MW01204421

EATING
MY WAY
TO
HEAVEN

Book Publishers Network

Book Publishers Network
P. O. Box 2256
Bothell, WA 98041
425 483-3040
sherynhara@earthlink.net

ISBN: 1-887542-23-X

Library of Congress Catalog Card Number:
98-073709

Manufactured in the United States
10 9 8 7 6 5 4 3 2

Editor: Vicki McCown
Cover Design: Bill Fletcher
Book Design & Production: Scott and Shirley Fisher

TABLE OF CONTENTS

Dedication i

In the Beginning There Was Steak 1

A Medium Is Born 9

"Puberty" Must Be Greek for "Hell".............17

From "Yous Guys" to Y'all"........................... 29

Flush 41

Rocky Mountain High 53

"Look, Mommy, It's the Karate Lady!"......... 65

Vince 81

Lowell 95

The Bodygaurd............................... 107

Stuck in Nevada Again........................ 119

CONTINUED

CONTENTS CONTINUED

Savvy! 137

Out on a Limb 153

The Magic Garden........................ 169

The Second Coming of Lowell 183

It Can't Be Denial...I Never Said That 199

The Sugar Detox Center 227

Travel Tales 247

Circles of Love 265

The Diary 273

DEDICATION

I lovingly, and with great appreciation,
dedicate this book to Patrick McEachern,
and Jocelyn Brewer.

Patrick helped me save my life, which you will read
about. And he agreed to let me share his less-than-
perfect behaviors, in service to the greatest good. But
most of all, he has put up with me as I have waded
through my old "baggage" trying to tell my story.
Thank you, Patrick!

Jocelyn spent three years poring over every word of this
book. Her genius with language has transformed my
story into a literary work.
Thank you, Jocelyn!

Many thanks to Joel Gallob,
Sybil Beale, and Vicki McCown for their edits and
literary input. Additionally, many thanks to all those
who invested monetarily, and/or with love and support,
to get me to market.

Thank you, Dr. Lendon (Dunny) Smith, for participating in our mission, for validating our beliefs, and for the
rich friendship you gifted me with. Rest in peace, Doc.
We'll take it from here. You are my hero!

And goodbye to another healthy-eating icon. I am proud to tell you that the delightful William Dufty (author, *Sugar Blues*) called me before he died. He beamed that he loved my book! It was a thrill for him to read about his impact on my life. Thank you, Dufty, for your deep sacrifices for the greatest good.

Most of all,
Thank you, God!

IN THE BEGINNING THERE WAS STEAK

My mother painfully admitted that I was an unplanned child. I wish I could ease her pain. That knowledge didn't hurt me. The fact that my father talked the doctor into inducing labor so that he could dash off on his hunting trip hurt me, especially since he loved to tell the story in my presence.

Karma kicked his butt, though. My mother ended up staying in the hospital for a week and he got to bring his new little bundle of joy home...alone! Mind you, he also had a four-year-old, a five-and-a-half-year-old, and a full-time job. My Aunt Eileen graciously helped out, but he still had plenty of alone time with his kids, which created the backdrop for his other favorite story.

Oh how he'd roar when he told this one at parties. He thought it made him appear quite ingenious. So did I, until a therapist pointed out with disgust that it had nothing to do with ingenuity.

David (my father) loved his sleep and had no intention of sacrificing any of it for a screaming, hungry newborn. When he was ready to go to bed he would heat me a bottle. If I dozed off while he was feeding me he would violently shake me awake until I had consumed the whole thing. He claimed that I always slept through the night.

This is a man who would lie down on the couch in the middle of the living room after dinner and state, "Wake me up when it's time to go to bed." The family's antics never woke him; neither did the biggest tornado to ever rock the East Coast. Chances are I had a number of wet, hungry, sleepless nights before my mother returned.

To my knowledge that was the last time that my father ever actively participated in feeding me, other than paying for groceries or meals in restaurants when we would travel.

For the record, I never called him "Dad" if I could avoid it. I spoke of him as my father and I have referred to him as David my entire adult life. To me, "Dad" describes a relationship we never had. David was a good provider, but not a dad.

He was always too busy or too uninterested to participate in my life, so I thought. I have come to realize that it had more to do with his emotional baggage than indifference. He had never gotten to be a kid, never gone away to camp or played with a neighborhood gang, and his mother had deserted him when he was very young.

Instead of wanting his children to have everything he never had, he wanted us to endure the same magnitude of suffering that he had endured. He thought it would build character and a healthy respect for work and money. It appeared that he had never healed his rage at his parents and we were convenient whipping posts.

We did eat well, though. David would complain as I would order steak or lobster from the menu, but ultimately he would relent and pay the bill. The underlying message was "Of course we love you; we feed you steak, don't we?"

Sweets and snacks were bargaining tools. "If you're good at church I'll buy you some candy." "If you eat all your dinner you can have some ice cream for dessert." Sugar became a subconscious symbol of "I am loved, I am good." That bears repeating. Sugar became a subconscious symbol of "I am loved, I am good."

The family rule was that you had to eat all the food on your plate or go to bed without dessert. I remember many evenings spent sitting over a cold plate of glop for hours (sorry, Mom), trying to get Duke's attention (my childhood best friend, our dog).

I learned to eat in large quantities to please my parents and I learned to love God in pursuit of my drug of choice – sugar! I looked forward to our pilgrimage to the candy store each Sunday after church. Actually, it wasn't really a candy store; it was a pharmacy, a drug store.

My brother, Sam, taught me how to turn a buck at a very young age. He was the consummate entrepreneur and I followed his lead. There was always a yard to rake, a driveway to shovel, or a lawn full of apples to pick up. Each new windfall prompted a manic trip to the candy store, pedaling as fast as my little legs could go. I would buy as much as I could afford or carry.

I tried to ration my booty, but even at the ripe old age of eight I was an out-of-control addict. Fortunately, I was so active that I stayed thin.

Halloween, of course, is the sacred holiday of sugar junkies. I worked it for all it was worth. I would usually come home with a half a pillowcase full of candy. My mother would ration it for us, so we got wise to her and stashed some of the candy in our secret fort before returning home.

Eventually my teeth started to give way. David made us pay him five dollars for every cavity and we were not allowed Novocaine. (Penance for our sins.)

What I learned from all this was that I had to keep the money rolling in to support my habit, and that there were some painful consequences to my addiction. None of that slowed me down though. I was hooked, a junk food "junkie!"

Mine wasn't the only household where I was force-fed. Like every neighborhood in Westchester, New York, ours had the consummate Italian family, the Andriolas. I deeply loved these people. The food thing had a different slant at the Andriolas.

Lois, Mrs. Andriola to me, spent her life in the kitchen. She'd clean up one meal and start another. When I rolled in to play with her sons she would always offer whatever was on the stove. God forbid you were already fed or full. She took it as a personal insult if you didn't eat what was offered. And it wasn't enough to politely accept a bite. You had to eat until you were nauseous. Her heart was full of love, but it seemed she could only express it with food. Lois died of complications from her obesity. She was a dear soul.

Then there were the Abers. God bless them. As if five children weren't enough, they always had another half dozen in tow because they had a baseball diamond in their back yard. They frequently ended up feeding me or driving me someplace or paying my way. I felt like a part of their family until the day I overheard Mrs. Aber complaining that my parents never invited her kids over to play because they didn't want to sacrifice their manicured lawn or have to pop for a meal.

It was the truth, but it hurt me deeply. (Worse than that, the Abers weren't invited to our house because they were Jewish.) From then on I tried to be invisible during meal times at the Abers. I could have lived without the meals, but I could not have survived without the Abers.

I was also force-fed at school. Once you forked over that lunch money to the commandant, you were locked in. They determined how much they piled on your plate and they patrolled the lunchroom to make sure you ate it all.

When my father was out of town my mother would treat us to pigs-in-the-blanket (little hot dogs baked inside biscuits), pizza, KFC or McDonald's. Guess it was her way of making up for David's behaviors, another subconscious symbol that food is more for our emotions or our entertainment than for nourishing our bodies.

So, let's recap. At my house and school you had to eat it all or you were in trouble. At the Andriolas' you had to eat until you were sick or offend someone you loved. And at the Abers' if you ate you were a burden to the family. The only common thread was that everybody rewarded me with sweets if they thought I deserved it, if I was good!

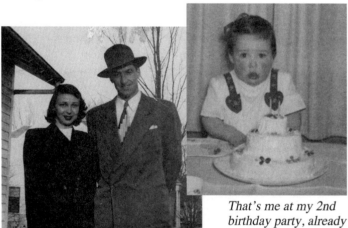

That's me at my 2nd birthday party, already deep in my sugar addiction. Check out those Rosacea cheeks!

My parents: David Moser and Patsy Ann Martin. Weren't they a dashing couple?

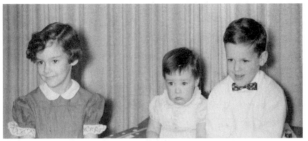

Paula, little Denise and Sam. My siblings were pretty darn cute.

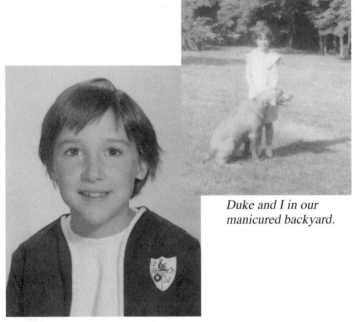

Duke and I in our manicured backyard.

Every day was a bad hair day with David and his bowl and scissors for my barber.

FOOD FOR THOUGHT...

The emotional roots of my food addiction seem pretty obvious to me. My parents weren't capable of warmth or demonstrative love. Sugary treats were the only display of affection that they could muster and their most powerful tool for control.

I hadn't considered that my sugar addiction might be hereditary. My father liked an occasional bowl of ice cream but really didn't seem to be too interested in sweets, and I don't recall that my mother had any driving need for them either, although they both indulged at an occasional social event. I now realize, though, that their daily consumption of alcohol was actually a sugar addiction, which I may have bio-chemically been born into.

What strikes me most, though, is that my parents knew refined sugar was bad. They rationed it to us and for themselves because they knew for sure that it rots our teeth and suspected that it was linked to many health problems. So how come they gave me something that they considered bad for me as a symbol that I was good? I imagine it was because the whole culture was doing it and they probably never even gave it a thought.

The social pressures connected with sugar and junk foods are quite vicious. We serve sugar at churches, schools, social events and holidays. Rarely is there a second choice. It's either have sweets or be left out. We have long forgotten how to celebrate without sugar or alcohol.

I remember my father being furious with us once because we had given our cousin Dick's horse some sugar cubes. David was booming, "You could kill him by feeding him that stuff!"

I didn't get it at the time, but it sure jumps up and screams at me now: "Here, Denise, have a candy bar, but for God's sake, don't give any to the horse. We don't want to lose him!"

Not everyone chooses sugar as their drug of choice. But for those who do, it is a very destructive love affair since it is everywhere, in everything and it's legal.

JUST FOR FUN...

Two cannibals are sitting by a fire. The first one says, "Gee, I hate my mother-in-law." The second one suggests, "So, try the potatoes!"

Taken from "The Edge" – The Oregonian, Portland, OR 11/1/97

A Medium Is Born

Although I lived in terror of my father, part of me really wanted a relationship with him. I rarely ever got to hang out with him unless he was drunk and we were pounding on the piano together. That only happened a few times a year (the piano thing, that is), but it was fun. It didn't matter that he couldn't sing worth a damn; he sang loudly instead.

David didn't play all that well, either, but as with his singing, he compensated with volume and it brought him great pleasure. "This Old House" and "How Great Thou Art" were his favorites.

A relative told me that my father was a deeply religious person before going off to war to serve as a Hell Diver in the South Pacific. They said that he was standing on street corners, straight out of college, preaching the Gospel. I had thought that religion was just a status thing for him. I never heard him talk about God or what it meant in his life unless he was speaking as an elder or deacon of the church. I did, however, sense his reverence for God when he sang "How Great Thou Art" — it moved him.

In recent years I have discovered that my mother is a very spiritual person and shares many of my beliefs, but I don't recall ever hearing her discuss God as I was growing up, either. Like most families, we went to church and that was it. We attended services every Sunday until we moved onto a golf course. Then, religious observance often gave way to tee times.

I was a very spiritual child but really didn't recognize it as such. I certainly didn't relate to the fear and damnation that the Sunday school teachers were cramming down my throat. But the minister of the Presbyterian Church we attended was a wonderful being who treated me with a lot of love and respect.

The real church for me, though, was just past the stone wall in our backyard. I was accutely in tune with the nature spirits I played with in the woods behind our house. My experiences in the woods were more than just those of a fanciful child playing make-believe. There was something out there that interacted with me, an energy that embraced me and made me feel loved and at home.

My other-dimensional playmates brought me a lot of comfort, as did the companionship of my fellow scouts. Being a Girl Scout provided me with a lot of rich experiences growing up. I especially treasured the opportunities to get away from home for a weekend of exploration or a few weeks during the summer to attend camp.

One particular campout changed my life forever. My spirituality crossed the line into the realm of the paranormal. The counselors sent home a very different child than the one they had received.

It was called a roundup. Girl Scouts came from all over New York, but I was the only one from my troop. As was customary for young girls at such gatherings, we decided to have a séance. What wasn't customary was to pick a subject to contact who invoked so much intrigue.

Pam Lacaruba wanted us to contact her grandfather. She said that her mother had been trying to contact him for years by hiring mediums. It seems that Pam's grandfather had changed his name and absconded with the family fortune before he died. Pam's mother wanted to find out what he had changed his name to so she could chase down her inheritance. Thus far she had been unsuccessful.

There were seven or eight of us sitting cross-legged in a circle as one girl led us into a deep meditative state. I don't remember her now, but as I pull up this memory I am impressed with what a mature storyteller she was at such a young age. We were all around the age of twelve or so.

Shortly after she started her litany, several things happened to me. I started feeling sharp pains in my fore-arms, my hands began to cramp and curl up, and visions were popping into my head. (Pam told me later that her grandfather had debilitating arthritis in his hands throughout his life.)

I began sharing my visions with the group, my eyes wide open most of the time. As I described the person and the home that I was seeing, Pam excitedly exclaimed, "That's my grandfather and that's his house!" These weren't educated guesses I was spewing out. I could describe the floor plan of the house, the arrangement of the furniture and the design of the wallpaper. I still remember some of the details to this day.

Not only could I describe Grandpa and emulate his arthritis, I was feeling his emotions. He and his deceased mother were acting out some cosmic play in my head. What I was sensing (which Pam's mother confirmed later) was that this had been a very abusive relationship between Grandpa and his mother. She had been wicked and mean. Also, I was perceiving that he had not seen her for many years previous to her passing on.

In my vision, Grandpa was experiencing a great deal of fear. He had a key in his hand and he was standing at the foot of a long staircase that led up to a locked door. Somehow I knew that when he opened that door he was going to be face to face with his mother for the first time since her death or his.

My heart raced a little faster with each step he took up the staircase. I had become Grandpa. If you're having a hard time swallowing this, believe me, I understand. I lived it and I am still incredulous every time I tell it, and it gets even more unbelievable!

When Grandpa opened the door at the top of the stairs I felt the most extreme terror I had ever experienced in my life. This evil-looking woman was standing there, oozing rage. I looked up at the innocent girl across from me and watched in horror as her face took on the countenance of the old woman, and I wasn't the only one who saw it. I screamed and jumped out of the tent, which was up on a platform about four feet off the ground.

I flopped around in the dirt like a fish out of water with my hands cramped up in knots as the rest of the girls stood and watched in horrified silence. One girl, Debbie Woods, went into shock. She seemed catatonic, with her eyes stuck open and a lit flashlight in her hand. She couldn't speak or move her gaze from the glow of the flashlight, becoming manic if someone tried to take it from her. We had to summon help. This was out of our league.

I came out of my shock and my "arthritis" abated, but Debbie was not coming around. The counselors took her somewhere to get her medical attention. When they returned we were cautioned to "Never do anything like this again" and, of course, "Forget this ever happened."

The rest of the weekend was uneventful, comparatively speaking. We returned to our respective homes, honoring the inflicted code of silence.

On Monday, I got a call from Pam Lacaruba's mother. She wanted me to come to their home for a séance (that's not what she told my mother). Come Friday, my mother drove me the thirty miles or so and deposited me for what she thought would be a weekend sleepover with a new friend. Twenty-five years later I told her the real story. She believed me to the best of her ability.

From the moment I walked in the door of Pam's house I was treated like royalty. After greetings and the offer of a beverage, I was walked to the dining room table. Pam's mother had covered the table with hundreds of photographs.

She said, "Show me what you saw."

I had no trouble picking out Grandpa, his mother and the house, describing the furniture and the wallpaper again in flawless detail. Mrs. Lacaruba declared, "Child, you have a gift!" As I recall she gave me a list of things to do to develop my psychic powers. I didn't do them and I don't remember what they were. I wish I did.

We went on to perform the séance. Mrs. Lacaruba was sure that I would be able to come up with the elusive name she was hunting for. Nothing happened. I felt bad for letting her down, but I imagine that I was too terrified to actively participate.

As the dutiful child I was, I buried the memory for the most part and went on with my life as if nothing had happened. But inwardly my entire belief system had been rattled.

FOOD FOR THOUGHT...

One belief has changed for me since then for sure. I no longer believe in accidents or coincidences. Here's an example of what some might consider a coincidence. You decide.

As I was editing this book, I had some doubts about whether any of the girls at that séance would remember it now that nearly thirty years have passed.

My fear was that if they didn't, it would cast doubt on the validity of all my memories. I was also concerned that they might have buried this traumatic memory, as often happens with children.

That same week a package came for me from my mother. There was no note or letter included, just a collection of a few mementos of mine from childhood. Amongst the items was an old autograph book. Back then young girls enjoyed gathering signatures and quips from friends. This particular autograph book was filled with entries from the girls at that roundup. Four of them mentioned the séance in their writings and one of them even drew a picture of what my arthritic hands had looked like. I was jubilant. It was the validation I'd craved.

My mother didn't know I had included that story in this book or that I was anxious about it. She was just cleaning out a drawer and thought I would like to have these things. Was it a coincidence? I don't think so. I think God, Great Spirit, the Universe – whatever your concept of a supreme power is – responded to my needs.

JUST FOR FUN...

Speaking of coincidences, renowned author and speaker, Alan Cohen, told this story when he spoke at the Living Enrichment Center in Wilsonville, Oregon. Alan is the author of thirteen books about living life fully, including my favorite, Are You As Happy As Your Dog? about his dog Munchie's joyous slant on life. In my words here is the story Alan told:

For Thanksgiving, Alan had put on a big spread for his mostly vegetarian friends. Someone, however, had brought a large turkey. It seems little Munchie was the major benefactor of that offering and feasted on turkey for a month. When the stash was gone Munchie had no intention of going back to his old diet of "little pellets." Alan noted, "It's like life. Once you've seen the big turkey, you won't want to settle for little pellets!" As a vegetarian though, Alan couldn't see himself trotting off to the market to buy a turkey, so he left it in God's hands.

A few days later, Alan was driving to his home in Maui and noticed a police car behind him in the mirror. He apparently hit a time warp in his mind and found himself stuck in sixties paranoia, frantically searching for non-existent contraband. He pulled himself together by reciting this affirmation, "The police are my friends, the police want to help me." The police car passed him up, not even noticing Alan.

One evening not long after, Alan pulled up to a police roadblock. It seems that they tip a few too many in Maui and the police department had come up with an incentive program to reward sober drivers. After chatting with Alan and inspecting his paperwork, the officer shouted, "Hey, Joe, come here." Alan had a bit of concern as to why this officer needed Joe, but recited his "the police are my friends" mantra and kept calm.

Joe leaned in the window of Alan's car and asked, "Do you want a turkey?"

Alan laughed, "Is this a joke?" Officer Joe explained that they were giving away turkeys to anyone whose paperwork was in order and who wasn't drunk. They only had six turkeys so apparently they weren't too confident they'd find many qualifying candidates that night. Alan had his picture taken with officer Joe and his frosty new Butterball and laughed all the way home.

Upon being greeted by Munchie, Alan proclaimed, "You are a great manifester. You got the police to give you a turkey!" Was it a coincidence or was it an answered prayer for Alan and Munchie?

"PUBERTY" MUST BE GREEK FOR "HELL"

Physically, I hit puberty at twelve, which was considered early in 1969. These days, little girls are sprouting breasts and menstruating at eight, thanks, in my opinion, to all the steroids and hormones in the dairy products and the meats.

Apparently, 1969 was not to be my year. Whether it was ghostly experience at camp, the new rush of hormones, my father's crap, I don't know, but this shaped up to be the worst twelve months of my short life.

Along with the new breasts (I'm talking puberty, not implants) came a boyfriend. Robby Moravec spent most of his energy trying to get his hands on the new breasts or get me in bed. He spent hours talking dirty to me on the phone every night. I don't remember why we broke up, but I do recall getting quite worn out on the sex talk and trying to fight him off. Interestingly enough, a few years later, I dated one of Robby's best friends, Robert Pastor. He eventually dumped me because I was too "fast" for him. I was frustrated because he was too shy to kiss me or even hold my hand. Go figure.

Boys weren't my only challenge at this point in my development; men were even worse. My father derived great pleasure from humiliating me in front of his friends, our neighbors. My descent into puberty furnished him with a plethora of new materials.

As I revisit those memories of him and his friends laughing at me over some demeaning comment he would make about my breasts, I wonder whether these men were really as cruel as my father was or just didn't want to risk offending him. David was a powerful man, a top executive for Texaco.

Each year, from the time I was twelve until I got my first real job at fifteen, my parents bought me a new winter coat, shoes and some boots. My mother, God bless her, would dip into the grocery money (David never knew) and buy material to sew me up some fabulous garments to supplement my wardrobe. She also popped for a few new store-bought items each fall.

Shopping was a very grown-up privilege that my parents had bestowed on me. They wanted to teach their children how to be responsible with money (a lesson that has been lost on me thus far). I was given twenty dollars a month to purchase the remainder of my wardrobe. But we also had other expenses for which we were accountable.

As kids, we were charged a nickel every time we left the room and left the light on, a dime for each outgoing phone call, and then there were those "five dollar per cavity" dental bills. I could spend what was left of my allowance on movies, candy or whatever. Rarely was anything left over. But I did odd jobs and babysat throughout my childhood, and so was able to keep the money rolling in fairly consistently.

Perhaps it was a good theory for fostering responsibility, but I think a child should concentrate on reading, writing, arithmetic and play, instead of pulling down a living to pay off Daddy.

Anyway, if I could get myself the five miles to downtown Valhalla, (my hometown, which I understood loosely means "Heaven" in Norse mythology), I could get on a bus and ride the twenty miles or so to White Plains to go shopping. I usually went with a friend whose mother would drive us to the bus stop. Sometimes my mother would drive us or we would walk.

On this particular day I went to White Plains with Nina, the most popular girl in the school. I had twenty dollars on me. I don't know how much she had, but I imagine it was at least that much.

We decided to steal something for the thrill of it. I stole a pair of socks. I think Nina lifted a bra. I remember standing in front of this post that had mirrors on all four sides. I was holding a sweater up to my chest and admiring it in the mirror. After stuffing our ill-gotten booty in our shopping bags we headed for the door. There was a young woman walking ahead of us who looked like something out of Laugh In with her mini-skirt and go-go boots, and an old woman walking behind us.

As soon as we stepped out the door, they grabbed us. They were undercover security officers for Alexander's Department store. I later found out that the mirrored posts were hollow. Security people stood in them to watch shoppers. And I thought I had been so clever the way I had been admiring that sweater in the mirror while I slipped the socks in my bag. To this day I can't seem to keep a decent pair of socks in the house — more karma I guess.

I experienced a level of terror that was even a step up from the séance. These women scared me, but that wasn't it. The six-foot-five store manager scared me, but that wasn't it. The threat of the police scared me, but that wasn't it either. I knew that eventually they would turn me over to my father. That scared the hell out of me. So, I did the only thing that I could think of in my terror — I lied. I gave them a false name, address and phone number.

Meanwhile, they were extracting information from Nina in a separate room. The woman who was questioning me walked across the hall to Nina and asked, "What's your friend's name?" I was toast.

The store manager was then called in to intimidate me. He said that he was going to call the police because I had lied and made matters worse. I think I told him that I would rather face the police than my father. So, of course, he called my father.

Amazingly, my parents seemed pretty calm. I was told that they were on their way to a football game. I was to take the bus home and wait for them in my room. It's incredible how time stands still sometimes. Perhaps it was the longest football game ever. It was certainly the longest day of my life.

As their car pulled into the driveway, my blood ran cold. They came to my room. I expected my father to be out of control with rage and fury. He wasn't.

My mother tried to get me to admit (attempting to help me I'm sure) that Nina had pressured me into doing this. God only knows why I chose that moment to find some integrity. I assured her that I was a willing participant, not a victim. I thought I'd score a few points with my father for that one. Apparently, I was too far behind in the game; any points I may have picked up did not impact the outcome.

David sat down on the bed next to me and began this calm, cool and collected speech. His oration included statements like I was the most disgusting person that he had ever met, and he was ashamed to be my father. I was grounded for a month, at which time we would reconvene to determine if I had learned anything from this experience.

I was in shock when they left my room. I thought, "What just happened?" I had expected a vicious beating or some time at the rock pile or something. Visions of

Sing Sing had danced through my head. Earlier in my childhood we had stopped to see Sing Sing, the infamous prison in Ossning, New York. I was petrified at the time that David would leave me there.

I vividly remember thinking on the day of my so-called arrest. "No matter what happens to me for the rest of my life, it will never be as bad as this day." So far, that has rung true. When times get tough I have had the comfort of thinking, "It's not as bad as that day!"

During the month of my sentence I wasn't allowed out of my room for anything except school and meals. My father ate in the living room, and we were fed in the kitchen. He felt that he shouldn't have to be bothered with children after a long day's work at the office, so I saw very little of him in that thirty days.

Being grounded was no big deal. I had plenty of toys and imagination and enjoyed playing by myself. I did the time with ease. At the end of the month, David came to my room. He asked if I had learned my lesson. I said, "Yes." I was paroled, or so I thought.

Some time passed before I actually noticed and registered what was going on. It was very subtle. If David passed me in the hall, he would look the other way. If I threw out a comment, he would ignore it. If I was out late babysitting, he would turn off all the lights and go to bed, never even checking to see if I got home safely. The cold war was on.

This continued until I went off to college six years later, with the exception of a handful of occasions. In all fairness to David, I will take a moment to tell you about those occasions, but first I must commend him on his ingenuity. By ignoring me he had inflicted on me the most painful punishment known to man, and I hadn't seen it coming. It was a setup to rob me of my self-esteem. For him I ceased to be as a person. Duke got more attention than I did. It hurt for decades!

During that six years I would feel physically nauseous while sitting in the same room with David. I also discovered alcohol and drugs shortly after my parole. Abandonment digs very deep.

My feelings about David were pretty extreme way before the shoplifting incident, though. I truly hated and feared my father. I can remember being eight and sitting in front of the TV watching the news when David was out of town. I was hoping to hear that his plane had gone down — pretty serious thoughts for an eight-year-old.

I also revered my father. He obviously was not cut out to be a parent, but he was outstanding in every other category of his life. He was a great businessman who demonstrated integrity, honesty and loyalty in business as well as in his friendships. He was a decorated war hero, a community leader, highly respected in the church and a darned hard worker. The fact that he was so cruel to me was especially hard to swallow when I had to watch him be such a stand-up guy to everyone else.

He did break down on a few occasions though and treat me lovingly. He came to my room one morning and barked, "Get dressed, we're going out." Man, I was scared. When we got in the car his tone changed.

I had wanted to take piano lessons for as long as I could remember. I watched enviously as my older sister, Paula, went off to her lessons. I loved to listen to her play. But David wouldn't let me take lessons because Paula had quit after six years, so I had taught myself to play.

Paula had a piano in her room. I'd ask her to show me which note was middle C and then I would follow the notes up the scale on the page with my finger as I advanced to the next note on the keyboard. I'm no Billy Joel, mind you, but I can read music and pound out "In the Garden" or "The Maple Leaf Rag" to my great delight.

During that unnerving car ride, David said that he had been wrong for not letting me take lessons just because Paula had quit. He also expressed that he was proud of me for sticking to it and teaching myself how to play. He took me to a piano store and told me to pick a brand new one. He paid cash for it and had it delivered.

Of course, the piano turned into a power struggle eventually – a gift with a million strings attached. But I am crying as I remember that brief moment of love he showed me.

My parents gave the coolest party every Fourth of July. They called it a Treasure Hunt. Fifty couples were invited to attend. It was the most talked-about event in their circle.

Two couples were paired up and given a cute, whimsical clue to start with. If they figured out the clue, it would take them to a spot somewhere in a five-mile radius of our house – a goal post at the high school, the flagpole at the post office, or something like that. There they would find a Texaco oil can with a new clue in it, until they got to the last location and clue that would lead them home. If they couldn't figure out one of the clues, they could call in for the answer, but would have twenty minutes docked off their time. The winning car received $100, $50 for second place. Then the eating, drinking and dancing would start.

Those were grand times for my parents. My father could be a real blast when he was looped. The code of silence was lifted each Fourth of July, and I truly enjoyed the bond I felt with him once a year.

There were two other occasions in my life (that I remember) when my father treated me with warmth and value. One was the week before we moved to Texas. My sister was off at college and my brother had run away from home (a long-established pattern for Sam by now).

David put his arm around me and apologized for being such a lousy father. He said that things would be different when we got to Houston. It would be my turn to be spoiled. Unfortunately, things got worse in Texas.

The other occasion was at the little country church that we attended, outside Houston, when David wasn't golfing. At fifteen I was a deacon in that church and got to be "Minister For A Day" one Sunday. I gave a sermon, played the guitar and sang, and was quite the little leader. My father beamed with pride and gave me some wonderful strokes. His feelings were sincere and were never retracted or used to manipulate me. That was heaven!

Anyway, back to hell, I mean puberty. I had one friend named Susan who seemed to be as miserable as I was. She was overweight and had deep family problems. Between the older boys she hung out with and my brother, we could usually get our hands on a bottle of whiskey.

Susan's parents would let us sleep in the camper in their driveway on weekends. We would hold our nose and chug that whiskey until the bottle was empty. We usually puked and passed out, but it was still a welcome reprieve from the emotional pain we were carrying.

My other friend, Nancy, who lived next door, was a year older than I. She ran with even older guys so she got her hands on marijuana and speed.

Nancy's mother was a wonderful loving person, sometimes. The rest of the time she was a falling-down drunk. She would come up to us on her hands and knees and beg for booze. It was pitiful.

One day Lois Andriola found Nancy's mother face down in the back yard in the snow. When Lois turned her over, a liquor bottle rolled out of her hands and she went crawling after it. Needless to say, Nancy had some emotions to sedate. So did I, especially after her mother took us on a wild, drunken ride home one afternoon from the swimming pool. I needed a drink by the time we pulled into the driveway.

It took me many tries to get high on pot, but the speed got me off the first time. I remember running up Greenwood Lane feeling like an Indian warrior. I could have run forever. I was a little scared, but I liked the feeling.

So let's see. At the advanced age of twelve I had a number of addictions to support. I still had my candy fetish (which stayed with me for another twenty-six years), I drank heavily on weekends, and I smoked pot and tried whatever hard drugs Nancy could rustle up. My brother told me then that he would kick my ass if he ever caught me smoking dope. A year later he was sharing his best weed with me.

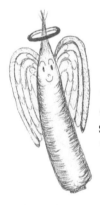

FOOD FOR THOUGHT...

It seems that people are getting tired of the abuse excuse because it has often been exploited in the courtroom. I argue both sides of the issues depending on which trial we might be discussing. I do think, however, that I have offered sufficient evidence to support my belief that I came by my addictions rightly. I take full responsibility for choosing to abuse sweets, alcohol and drugs, but the alternative was to cope with all these emotions straight, alone and without a crutch. I couldn't do it, especially in puberty.

My mother and I had a conversation about drugs a few years ago. It was her belief that kids try drugs looking for a thrill and then get hooked. I disagreed. I believe that a child who is loved and nurtured can go for a joy ride with drugs and walk away. It is those of us who are trying to use drugs, sex, money, work, whatever to fill the hole in our hearts who get hooked. The answer is more love, more love, more love.

I think that we need to stop raging at and blaming troubled teens for their behaviors. Let's try to help them through this difficult time. Puberty is when we really start to develop a sense of ourselves as a person. The shift in hormones can cause great physical turmoil along with all the emotions that arise concerning the passage out of childhood.

We accept that women have major mood swings because of the rise and fall of our hormones each month, but we don't give adolescent children any slack when their bodies are being hammered by hormonal shifts. I believe that the support we give children throughout puberty is one of our greatest tools for raising happy, healthy adults.

JUST FOR FUN...

On the subject of stealing...

A burglar broke into a house one night. He shone his flashlight around, looking for valuables. When he picked up a CD player to place in his sack, a strange, disembodied voice echoed from the dark saying, "Jesus is watching you." The burglar nearly jumped out of his skin, clicked his flashlight off, and froze. When he heard nothing more after a bit, he shook his head, clicked the light back on, and began searching for more valuables.

Just as he pulled the stereo out so he could disconnect the wires, clear as a bell he heard "Jesus is watching you." Freaked out, he shone his light around frantically, looking for the source of the voice. Finally, in the corner of the room, his flashlight beam came to rest on a parrot. "Did you say that?" he hissed at the parrot.

"Yep," the parrot confessed, "I'm just trying to warn you."

The burglar relaxed. "Warn me, huh? Who the hell are you?"

"Moses," replied the parrot.

"Moses," the burglar laughed. "What kind of stupid people would name a parrot Moses?"

"Probably the same kind of people who would name a Rotweiller Jesus," the bird answered.

An Internet jokester

From "Yous Guys" to "Y'all"

The three years following the Alexander's incident are pretty much gone from my memory. I don't remember most of my teachers or classmates. I recall little or nothing about the sports I played or the activities I participated in. I can't even remember any crushes or boyfriends I had, other than the "too shy to hold hands" guy, Robert. I walked through those years an empty shell.

In the middle of my freshman year of high school in New York, I was informed that we would be moving to Houston, Texas. David had been asked to develop a safety division for Texaco. To his credit, I recall his being quite overwhelmed by the whole thing. He admittedly knew nothing about the department he was about to create and head up. But as the consummate professional that he was, he ended up doing a stellar job. In later years I found the courage to master many projects that were out of my league. I thank my father for that courage. As you can see, the love/hate relationship I had with him has been the source of much of the turmoil in my life.

My parents had decided to wait until the end of the school year to make the move so as not to disrupt my studies. I was anxious to go, considering my father's heartfelt comment about how I would be spoiled in Texas. I spent many nights dreaming of the horse he would buy me and the beautiful country estate we would live on. I thought a change of venue would change my life. Oh it did, but it wasn't exactly what I had envisioned.

We ended up living in a very pretty place on a championship golf course. Fabulous, if you happened to be sixty or better and have a wardrobe of plaid pants and fire-engine-red sweaters. Not exactly a teen haven.

I made one friend in Texas before I ever even left New York. My parents had gotten Susan White's name and address from the real estate agent. We became pen pals. Her family lived just a few blocks from our new house.

Our first day at the house, we found that the furniture hadn't shown up yet (it was basking in the Kentucky bluegrass or someplace), so my parents decided to go off to the nursery to get some shrubs and plants. They left me behind at the house.

The temperature was a moderate 110 degrees, typical for August in Houston, as I was to find out. I was standing in the backyard (which actually was the rough of the fifth fairway of Champions, one of the top golf courses in the country) when a golf ball came flying into the yard, barely missing the wall of windows on the back of the house. Not knowing squat about golf, I picked up the ball and chucked it back onto the fairway.

A few minutes later, here came Mickey Rooney, in the most ridiculous outfit I have ever seen, looking for his ball. He was quite pleased to discover where his shot had landed (with a little help from a friend). I was thinking, "Cool. The first person I met in Texas is a movie star. This place is gonna be a blast!"

A little while later I noticed a whole group of black men coming down the fairway with golf bags slung over their shoulders. I burst out laughing. My father was the most bigoted person I'd ever met. I thought, "Wait til David sees the neighborhood he bought into. This is great!" It turned out that on Mondays they would let the caddies play the course.

My next encounter was with Agnes Weeren, the real estate agent. She was a pip and as pure Texan as they come. Agnes had the beehive hairdo, that wonderful knack for hospitality they all seem to share, and the thickest drawl I have ever heard. My mother used to joke, "How do you make a three syllable word out of Pat?" (Pat is my mother's name.)

Although I haven't seen Agnes since I was a teenager, I hear she still circulates this story too. I don't know if I can do it justice on paper, but I'll give it a go.

My parents had gone to Texas to house hunt without me, and apparently Agnes had gotten the impression that they didn't have any children (my siblings were no longer living at home). That first day in Texas, while I was alone at the house, Agnes stopped by. She introduced herself and asked me my name. I replied, "Denise."

She noted, "That's (pronounced "they ats") nice honey, but what's your naa…yah…mmm?" (Another three syllable word.)

I repeated, "Denise."

"I see, but what's your na…yay…mmm, huh…ney?"

I didn't speak the language. After some further discussion I finally deduced that she thought I was trying to relate to her that I was their niece. And so it began.

That was my first day in Texas. Besides being scorched by the heat, I had concluded that my father had bought a house on the wrong side of the tracks, met a movie star, and was now convinced that I was in a foreign land, unable to communicate with the natives.

Other than Agnes, the real problem wasn't the accent or semantics (Y'all every other word instead of Yous Guys), it was the pace that was the biggest problem. I spoke so fast that they didn't have a clue what I was talking about, and they talked so slowly that I didn't have the patience to hang around for the end of the thought.

In time my parents returned and the furniture arrived. We began the task of getting settled into our new home. A few days later I met Susan White face to face.

I was excited about meeting Susan. I had developed quite a fondness for her through our correspondence and a phone call or two. She, too, was a native with a southern drawl, but hers was adorable, not impossible to decipher.

By this time, puberty and my sugar addiction were taking their toll on me. I was a little overweight, had short, uncooperative hair, mild acne and my self-esteem was in the dirt. The new breasts were quite large now, offsetting my excess weight a bit, but I would have gladly traded them in for a size-four body and clear skin.

When my mother showed Susan into my room, I stared. Son-of-a-bitch if she wasn't drop-dead gorgeous. Susan was tall and thin. She had porcelain skin with just the right splash of freckles and legs that went on for miles. Goody. If that wasn't bad enough, she was so sweet that I couldn't find it in my heart to hate her. God knows I tried. Worse still, she was aspiring to go to modeling school.

I had a knack for befriending the most beautiful girls in the school. It must have been a manifestation of that invisible me that had ceased to "be." Try hanging out on a Friday night with two or three of the most beautiful females on the planet and see how much attention you get. Actually, the guys gave me a lot of attention. They wanted inside tips on how to get in so-and-so's pants. Instead, I ran interference for my friends and began my career as a caretaker/bodyguard.

Cindy Sempe and Kathy Abbott were two of the most stunning females I have ever met. We all sang in the choir and hung out together. Cindy had black, silky hair down to her butt, gigantic brown eyes, a tiny little body and a radiant smile. Kathy Abbott had thick, blond hair down past her waist, enormous "come hither" blue eyes and a body like Pamela Anderson's (except Kathy's breasts were real).

They both sang like birds. I sang okay. I was the smart one, the funny one, the tough one. Much as I wanted to hate them too, I loved them. I learned a lot by hanging out with them. I would have lopped off my right arm to look like either of them, but their beauty did have its price.

They were a lay, or a trophy, that almost every male wanted to score. Some of the really cool guys they were interested in never even asked them out, evidently suffering from the "she'd never go out with me" complex. Cindy and Kathy were rarely admired for their wit, their talents or their opinions. The guys couldn't see past their physical beauty and the girls hated them for it.

As if Susan, Cindy and Kathy weren't bad enough, Farrah Fawcett's family lived down the street. I vividly remember my father remarking one day, in my presence of course, "Her parents are so lucky to have such a beautiful daughter."

Despite the fact that I had a lot of firsthand knowledge about the pitfalls of beauty, I still believed it would gain me my father's approval. I'm no ugly duckling, by the way, but admittedly a notch or two down the scale from Farrah, Susan, Cindy or Kathy.

I was a good student, aspiring to go to medical school. I sang in the top choir in the state, designed a lab manual for the science department, played the piano and the guitar, played a number of sports well, and was the youngest assistant manager that Big H Fried Chicken ever had. It seemed that none of that stacked up against Farrah's beauty. That comment did more to drive my addictions and my eating disorders than any other event in my life. It stayed with me like a record with a scratch, playing endlessly in my head, for twenty-five years.

When Farrah made a couple of questionable appearances on late-night TV a few years back, the tabloids claimed that she was high on cocaine and crucified her. I felt guilty for wishing her ill all those years, and finally let it go. I'm sorry Farrah; it wasn't your fault.

Farrah obviously has aged gracefully. I can't help but wonder how Susan, Cindy and Kathy have fared. I sincerely hope that they are all healthy, happy and as beautiful as Farrah. But now that I am sleek, with clear skin and long hair, I have to admit that it would be poetic justice to find them all overweight and saggy, with bobbed haircuts.

Halfway through my first year in Texas, which was my sophomore year of high school, came another of those life-altering events. I was told that I would be participating in a fund-raiser for the choir. They handed me a box of those oversized chocolate-almond bars to sell, twenty-five pounds of them. That is akin to giving an ounce of cocaine to a coke addict to sell for charity and saying, "Now don't do any." Yeah, right! I may have sold a bar or two to my parents or a neighbor, but should the truth be known, it is my recollection that I devoured the bulk of them.

Having to pay for the chocolate bars out of my own pocket was nothing compared to the twenty-five pounds I put on, the vicious acne I got, and the negative emotional roll it put me on. With each pound I gained my father became more distant. He was dreaming of a child who looked like Farrah Fawcett; I was not even close to measuring up. He not only didn't speak to me (a long-standing habit by now), his energy reeked with disgust.

My mother turned me on to saccharin and my father made little remarks to try to curtail my eating. If I ate too much or reached for a snack, he made some snide comment. If I skipped a meal, my mother would insist I eat. I couldn't win.

I truly believe they meant well. They knew my being overweight in college and in the work force would hold me back, but their efforts just made matters worse. I did more drugs, more alcohol and more junk food. I turned to God, that ever-present voice that had guided me through childhood, that love and presence that I could always count on. I prayed and prayed. The voice had stopped. The presence was gone.

I got angry with God. I raged at him, "How could I have ever believed in you? A loving God would not let children be treated the way I have been treated. A loving God would not ignore the call of a desperately lonely teenager. How dare you abandon me now!"

I became an atheist and entertained thoughts of suicide. It was as if I had this little devil standing on my shoulder who kept a constant, negative, running dialogue going; a litany of my father's voice and my own, expounding the shortcomings of Denise. I couldn't stop that voice and I couldn't hear God's. But apparently God could still hear mine. He sent my brother home. I had an ally.

Just before we had moved to Houston, Sam had run away from home. He had made it to California and found work as a chauffeur for a wealthy doctor. Once back in Houston, Sam rented a small house, which I helped him decorate. We painted a mural in the bathroom, shellacked the kitchen walls with old newspapers, plastered black light posters everywhere and filled the waterbed. It was our oasis. Just as the last can of paint was being drained, Sam got busted. He was arrested for possessing half a joint of marijuana.

The district attorney gave Sam two choices — go to jail or join the Air Force. After we finished white-washing the freshly decorated house, Sam headed off for Lackland Air Force Base in San Antonio, Texas, after doing time (apparently they call it boot camp) in Biloxi, Mississippi. I felt abandoned again. I fell deeper into hell.

My last two years of high school are pretty much a blank. I'm sure the shrinks and psychologists would have a lot to say about this. My read on it is: If you spend every waking moment hating yourself to the core of your being, who the hell wants to remember it!

When I went back to Houston eighteen years later, Sam was really hurt that I couldn't remember most of the fun times we had shared. All I could remember was that I had two best friends my junior and senior year: Susan Pugh and Steve Fischer. I had a couple of memories of Susan, but considering that we had been inseparable for two years, they were few. She was now working in the oil industry.

Steve had become a prominent doctor and was married to a psychiatrist. I was terrified the day my sister-in-law took me to see Steve at his office. I was afraid that I wouldn't recognize him. He looked familiar, but if I had run into him on the street I wouldn't have had a clue who he was, even though physically he hadn't changed much based on his old high school pictures.

Over dinner that night, his wife asked me what I remembered about Steve. I said that I remembered that we had been lab partners for nine months and hung out nearly daily for two years but I had no memories of those times. Steve showed me a movie that he and I and a bunch of our friends had made together. I had no memory of it and didn't recognize any of the people. We were both stunned.

High school had not been the "time of your life" for me. I worked long hours and spent a lot of time on my studies and my artwork. I never attended a prom, a homecoming dance or a single school social. I slept with older men who used me for sex after pumping me full of drugs.

Besides its oppressive weather, the language barrier, and my horrible life there, Texas had a few other drawbacks. The bugs were the size of small dogs, the snakes were big enough to saddle and the humidity caused you to sweat like a pig the moment you walked out the door. The way I usually describe my run in Texas is that I died and went to hell for five years. (No offense intended towards those who love Texas. It just didn't work for me.)

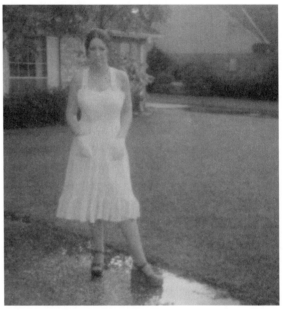

Me at my heaviest (high school graduation). I thought that I was too fat to walk the planet.

FOOD FOR THOUGHT...

What happened to me as a result of bingeing on chocolate was not unique. We now know that refined sugars depress the immune system and often our mental health and our spirits as well. It is the sudden swing of the hormones (insulin) to balance the sugar in our blood that can actually trigger anger, violence, a psychotic incident, depression, Attention Deficit Disorder and more. (Sugar spelled backwards is ragus – rages us!)

I wasn't really given a choice about selling the candy bars or I would have declined. I knew I couldn't control my addiction. Let's get kids and teens out selling earth-friendly products for fund-raisers, instead of having them peddle this highly addictive substance for cash.

Without a doubt, sugar was a gateway drug for me. If we want to fight the war on drugs we have to look at the reasons that kids get hooked, and address them, regardless of the legality (or not) of the substance they choose. More love, more love, more love is the answer.

JUST FOR FUN...

On the lighter side… In tribute to plaid pants and fire-engine-red sweaters, this is a good spot for a golf joke. Reverend Mary Manin Morrissey, founder of the Living Enrichment Center in Wilsonville, Oregon, slipped this one into a recent sermon.

Jesus and Moses were playing a round of golf. When they came to a particularly long hole, Jesus pulled out a seven iron. Moses tried to convince him to use a wood for this drive.

"Nonsense, if Tiger Woods can do it, so can I." Jesus drove his ball into the water.

"I'll get it," Moses said, and he parted the water and retrieved Jesus' ball.

Jesus wanted to try the drive again. Again he pulled out his seven iron, and again Moses suggested he use a wood.

"Nonsense. If Tiger Woods can do it, so can I." Jesus drove his ball back into the water.

This time Jesus muttered, "I'll get it." He walked across the water, reached down and fetched his ball.

Meanwhile, a foursome had come up behind the pair and witnessed this last scene. One of the golfers said to Moses, "Who does he think he is, Jesus Christ?"

"No," replied Moses, "he thinks he's Tiger Woods!"

FLUSH

I chose Austin College in Sherman, Texas, (sixty miles north of Dallas) because it had a great reputation for pre-med, and partially because it was a dry town (no alcohol served there). I thought it would keep me from drinking. As my teen-age friends would say, "Not!" It was a short walk across campus to find a fraternity bathtub full of Everclear (pure grain alcohol) that someone had driven the thirteen miles to Oklahoma to get.

Once again, I thought a change of venue would change my life, and once again, it did. Another giant step backwards.

Although I had always been a straight-A student in math, I flunked calculus my first semester, apparently not my cup of tea. Though I had managed to squeak through chemistry in high school, it was now a monster also.

Besides my studies I had a couple of other teensy-weensy challenges. I had no money, so I had to sling hash at Denny's on the graveyard shift. I had no wheels to get there with, no time to study. And I broke my right arm, so I couldn't write.

My classmates, who were some of the thousands of applicants I would be competing against to get into medical school, seemed to be well funded. I was not. The reason I was broke, however, was a bigger issue than the fact that I had no money.

Not long after Sam returned to Houston, I had come home from school one day to find him and my mother waiting for me at the door.

"We're going to the bank," my mother stated.

Somehow this didn't feel like a good thing. I wasn't sensing that we'd won the lottery or had received a visit from Publishers Clearing House. Apparently my brother was in some sort of trouble. My mother wanted to eliminate the problem without my father finding out. It required money. I was told, not asked, to give the $1000 I had in my savings account to Sam.

I was a sophomore in high school at the time, saving for college. I dreamed of being a thoracic surgeon. I loved my brother. We had always run interference for one another and I wanted to help, but I also wanted to realize my dream.

"Okay, I'll do it, but I want the money back before I go to college." They agreed, but it wasn't until twenty years later that I would get my $1000 back.

I could have earned more money before college except that my father made me quit my job at Big H Fried Chicken not too long after Sam wiped out my savings. David said that I was spending too much time at work and good grades for college were more important.

When I went to college, my father paid my tuition, but I had no money for books, supplies, shampoo, tampons, snacks, anything. I tried to get a student loan, but because my father made so much money I wasn't eligible. I had no choice but to get a job, hence, Denny's.

Now for my broken arm excuse: My brother had been quite good on the trampoline and I pretty much did everything he did. Though I wasn't as good as Sam, I wasn't bad. I was unofficially coaching some students at Austin College on the trampoline, as I had the most experience. I taught them how to catch by locking their arms in front of their chest. If someone were to come flying off the trampoline towards them they could block with their forearms and keep the person from leaving the mat. One day one of the guys participating in our trampoline group came back from swimming practice very tired. My intuition was to tell him to wait for another day. I ignored my inner voice.

He did a couple of sloppy layouts (a three-quarter back flip that lands you on your belly) and started another one. He ended up flying off the trampoline towards me. He was destined to land on his back on the bars and then tumble to the floor. Instead of doing what I had taught everyone to do, I panicked and threw my hand up and hurled him back onto the mat. I sensed that something was very wrong, but I felt no pain.

When I looked down, my wrist was about an inch around, all my bones were in a pile and my fingers were sticking out at a ninety-degree angle. They aren't designed to go that way! I freaked out and took off running. My fellow gymnasts caught up with me and treated me for shock. I was taken to the hospital.

I wanted a local anesthetic, but the doctor insisted on giving me general anesthesia, which meant that I had to spend the night. To my knowledge, I had never spent the night in a hospital before. I slept soundly after the surgery until about 2 a.m. when a nurse came in and woke me to ask if I wanted a sedative to help me sleep.

I barked, "I was sleeping fine. No, I don't want any drugs. Why did you wake me up?"

Now I found myself wide-awake. After several sleepless hours I called her back demanding that she "Bring me some Demerol!" She did, and they triple-charged me for it. This was the first of my many experiences with the corrupt medical profession I thought I wanted to join.

Tips at Denny's picked up significantly as I waited tables with my wrist to shoulder cast. There's nothing like a little plaster to open up those wallets. My studies didn't flourish, however; my grades were pretty dismal.

When my quarterly report card reached my father's desk, I was summoned home to explain my grades. Instead, I stalled, saying I couldn't get away from my classes for a few weeks. I was hoping for an earthquake or a nuclear attack or something that would save me from this meeting with my father. Although I seemed to be an expert at manifesting disasters, nothing happened. So I had a nervous breakdown instead.

Faced with the looming encounter with my parents, I didn't sleep for seven days. My mind and body were breaking down. So I grabbed three of my roommate's stomach tranquilizers, in keeping with my lifelong theory that if one is good, three times the recommended dose must be better.

I slept like a baby for ten hours or so. When I woke up I stumbled to the dormitory bathroom. I was splashing water on my face when I realized that I was blind. I couldn't see my own reflection in the mirror or my hand when I held it up to my face. I was also so desperately thirsty that I couldn't get two feet away from a water fountain without having to go back for more water.

My roommate got me to the campus infirmary. The nurse there noted that temporary blindness and severe dehydration were the side effects of overdosing from these pills, according to the Physician's Desk Reference. And they weren't all that convinced on the temporary part. I was scared. Fortunately, they agreed that involving my parents would not help the situation, as they were the source of my anxiety. In a few days my vision returned and my thirst backed off.

I still had to go face David, though. I now had my sister's car, which I had hitchhiked to Iowa to get. I was to deliver it to New York for her in a month or so.

I was exhausted by the time I got in the car to drive the three hundred miles from Sherman to Houston. I had attended school that day and then worked all night. I picked up a box of No-Doze for the drive.

I popped the No-Doze (which contains concentrated doses of caffeine) like M&M's the whole way. I was so buzzed that I pulled into my parents' driveway, stepped out of the car and fell to the ground.

"Oh this is going well," I pronounced loudly to myself.

Soon I was standing in the den like a war criminal facing a firing squad. My parents were somber and seated. I explained that my job and my broken arm had interfered with my ability to maintain my grades. My father wanted to know why I was working. Where had all my money gone?

My choices were to betray my mother and brother's secret or to take it in the shorts for something that wasn't my fault. I took the heat. I told him that I had squandered it.

I listened to an endless verbal assault about my stupidity and headed back to school the next day. A few months later, about to flunk a final exam, I decided to bag the whole college thing and move back to New York, where Paula was.

Once in New York, even with 2000 miles between us, I about collapsed when I called my parents to tell them that I had left school. I don't remember any of that conversation.

It felt good to have Paula's support, but we hardly knew each other. It had been six years since we had lived together on Greenwood Lane in Valhalla, New York. She had left home to go to college when I was twelve. There is a big gap between twelve and eighteen. We didn't have much of a relationship then, nor did we stay in close contact after she went off to school.

Of course Paula had the right to go to college, but my twelve-year-old mind hadn't registered that. All I knew was that she had left me there with them, and I had never really forgiven her for that.

Now, six years later, we were reunited. We didn't know each other at all as adults. She was about to undertake twenty years of being my surrogate mother, shouldering this burden out of guilt, because she had dared to leave home to go to college and leave me in an abusive situation.

Shortly after I arrived in Albany, Paula and her boyfriend Teddy took me out to their neighborhood watering hole for a drink. Teddy and I each ordered a glass of beer. Paula had her usual Canadian Club and gingerale. When Teddy went to the bathroom, I turned to Paula and stated, "When Teddy comes back I think I'll ask him if he wants to chug a beer for a buck."

She remarked, "Oh, he drinks a lot of beer."

"So do I," I told her. She didn't know that Sam had gotten me a false Canadian I.D., which enabled me to get into bars at fifteen. (I spoke enough French to pull it off.) She also didn't know that Sam had taught me to chug pitchers of beer. I was good!

When Teddy came back I challenged him to a chugging contest. The loser was to buy the winner another beer and a shot of Tequila and pay one dollar. He laughed and put his dollar on the bar. Paula would be the official timekeeper. When she gave the signal I hoisted my mug, poured the beer down my throat and returned the mug to the bar in my usual time – two seconds.

Teddy had not even taken a single sip from his glass. He was stunned. Thus began my career as a professional drinker. Every guy in town had to challenge me after the word got out. Nobody could beat me, so they nicknamed me "Flush."

I could go out every night, drink until I puked and come home with a profit. One night I was so drunk that I ended up lying on the bathroom floor of the bar at 4 a.m. They were trying to close up, but the room was spinning too fast for me to get up and leave. I told the bar owner to just lock me in, promising not to touch anything. Of course he wouldn't. It became apparent that it was time for me to get a life.

Unfortunately, that wasn't the last occasion that my drinking got out of hand. There was the time I went to a party with Paula and Teddy, deeply depressed because I couldn't find any work. I spent most of the time by myself drinking wine.

Later, I was walking down a steep hill in the dark, towards a lake, looking for a tranquil spot in which to continue my "Oh poor me" roll. I stumbled and fell and ended up face down in the water. I remember lying there in the water thinking that my arm was broken, but I never made any attempt to pull my head out so I could breathe.

I must have made quite a commotion during my drunken tumble, because Paula and a few others came running. She thought I was dead as she lifted my head out of the water. She was so traumatized by the event that I quit drinking for a while. Alcohol was one of the few substances that I could walk away from at will, because it was fattening and often made me sick. I preferred drugs.

I took the last of my money, moved out of Paula's trailer and rented a room in a boarding house. I had twenty dollars left for food. I stocked the little kitchen I shared with an old man and the young guy down the hall. The old guy would try and pour whiskey in my milk when I wasn't looking, and the young guy ate all my food, even though he made twenty-five dollars an hour working for the railroad. I just couldn't seem to turn things around.

One day I saw an ad in the paper for the job of my dreams. A new dinner theatre was opening in Albany. They were looking for people who could sing, dance and wait tables. I really didn't believe that I was good enough, but I went for it anyway.

It was slated to be an old English dinner theatre. When I called about the auditions, they told me that I should show up prepared to sing the tune of my choice – a cappella. I spent days in front of the mirror practicing "Loverly" in my best cockney accent. I really didn't expect to get the job, but on the other hand, I planned to be devastated if I didn't.

When the auditions started, they asked for a volunteer to go first. I threw my hand in the air. I could tell that they were in a hurry, so I thought that jumping out of my chair would score me some points. To my horror though, they stopped me halfway through my song. I was about to go into a manic depressive roll when the woman running the auditions said, "You're hired," then turned to the rest of the applicants and announced, "That's the kind of talent we're looking for." They didn't need the best of Broadway, just people who could carry a tune, a tray and some exuberance for a few hours a night. I was in heaven!

Trouble was, I had no food and no money with several weeks of rehearsals to go before ever seeing a tip or a paycheck. I moved in with one of the other girls from the show, but she had no more money than I did. So, we set up an account with the local mom-and-pop grocery store down the street. They let us charge up a jar of peanut butter here, a pack of cigarettes there. When we'd get really low on smokes, we'd pluck all the butts out of the garbage can, dump the tobacco out and roll a fresh cigarette. If there weren't enough butts we'd just smoke the ones we had down to the filter.

I loved the job at the dinner theatre. I learned the dance numbers quickly, so the choreographer had me teaching the others at times. Finally, a little self-esteem was creeping into my life. Not for long, however. The show packed up for Miami in a few months and I was not one of the chosen few invited to go on the road.

About this time, my sister hosted a reunion of a bunch of her old buddies from around the country. I ended up having laryngitis the weekend that they all showed up. I could barely gravel a word. Tom, one of Paula's closest friends, had traveled from Colorado for the reunion. He and I fell in lust. We spent the whole weekend together without my uttering a word above a whisper. After he returned to Denver we wrote long, mushy letters almost daily. It seemed we had fallen in love. He was nearly six years older than I, and 2000 miles away, but that didn't seem to matter.

In the meantime, Faith had come into my life, a woman with two children who lived in the ghetto. She was quite functional when it came to dealing with the government in an effort to get her welfare, but she had never known anything else. A continuous stream of welfare checks and food stamps was as big as she could dream.

I went to visit her one night in the ghetto. Her very large, very abusive boyfriend was there. This guy reeked trouble. Faith indicated that there was a warrant out for his arrest for seven counts of armed robbery.

Her adorable little girls were about three and five. Steve, the boyfriend, was calling Faith a whore in front of her kids. To this day I don't know what came over me. I picked up an ice pick and told him to leave. He stared me down for a moment and decided that maybe I was crazier than he was. He left. I became the new head of this brood.

Faith had leukemia and couldn't care for these children on her own, so I moved in. I had taken a job as a caregiver making $100 a week. I paid the rent of $100 a month, my car payment, insurance, the electric bill, and tried to put food on the table. Somedays I had to steal food to get everybody fed. Faith ate first, then the kids. The stray dog and cat and I fought over the leftovers.

I slept on the couch with a spring sticking in my back. The kids slept on a bare mattress, they each had a sheet. Faith had a bed with one blanket. We had an ice pick stuck in each door jam for security. We used the stove to heat the place, and after the toilet blew up we had to squat outside. It was definitely not heaven!

A friend of Faith's named Phyllis Frey showed up from Massachusetts with a boyfriend in tow. They couldn't find work right away, so I was now feeding four adults, two children and two animals. We lived on potatoes, ramen and bread. I dropped a few pounds but I was still about twenty pounds overweight and suffering from malnutrition.

Phyllis was about forty pounds overweight and one tough biker chic, but I liked her. We forged a bond that lasted for seven years. To this day, I consider Phyllis the best female friend I have ever had. She taught me about honesty and friendship. Her boyfriend left before long and it was just us gals.

I was scared to death of getting stuck in the ghetto. My father had been traumatized by the Depression and held tightly to the fear of poverty. I thought that if I didn't get out soon, it would become a lifetime struggle of trying to break free. I was saving my pennies to move to Colorado to be with Tom, planning to take Faith and the kids with me.

Instead, Faith fell in love with a medical student from NYU and decided to stay behind, so Phyllis planned to join me instead. I had lost my car to the bank after getting behind on the payments. Phyllis and I saved a few dollars and set out to hitchhike to Colorado — anything to get out of the ghetto.

The change-of-venue theory was working so well for me that I decided to give it another shot. It was a pretty good gamble that things couldn't get worse. On to Colorado...

FOOD FOR THOUGHT...

It was a real eye opener for me to be living in extreme poverty after the abundant life I had experienced as a child. The most startling discovery for me was to see that Faith's children were happy! They only had a few toys but we all put a lot of energy into playing and talking with them. Faith didn't have any money to provide them with a comfortable life, but she was by their side, all day, showering them with love and strokes. They were much happier than I had been, living in the luxury of Westchester, New York.

Perhaps that is one of the messages that I picked up along the way that caused me to choose poverty for so many years, thinking it was a noble gesture.

My work in the dinner theatre was fun, but the applause didn't have much effect on my infinitesimal self-esteem. I could barely hear the applause over the thunder of my inner demons screaming for my attention. All I could do was keep acting out, hoping somebody would eventually save me from myself.

JUST FOR FUN...

In tribute to my brief stint in show business, I'll share one of my favorite jokes from childhood.

There was a sweet old man named Jake who worked for the circus. Day in and day out for fifty years he had followed the elephants around and cleaned up after them, furiously shoveling away.

One day his close friend, Abe, approached him and said, "Jake, why don't you retire and enjoy the fruits of your labor? You've earned it."

Without missing a shovelful, Jake exclaimed, "What, and give up show biz!"

Rocky Mountain High

Phyllis and I did a lot of hitchhiking during our friendship. We became quite the team. We were some place in Pennsylvania, on our way to Colorado, when a drunken old man picked us up. Before long he was making crude comments.

Listening to sexually offensive come-ons by men is sometimes the nature of the beast when hitchhiking, but this guy crossed the line. He looked at me and said, "Well, maybe I'll just rape you."

Before I could even formulate a response, Phyllis pulled out a big buck knife and raged, "Well, maybe we'll just kill you and take your truck! Now pull over, you @#$%!" I didn't know her well enough to know if she was bluffing or not, but he believed her!

Hopefully, I've already talked you out of ever hitchhiking. Suffice it to say, you'd better be as tough as Phyllis or I before you ever consider putting your thumb in the air. Even then, it's a serious gamble. Rape and murder aren't the only dangers of jumping in with strangers either.

One time I was hitchhiking in Houston when an older man in a brand new Cadillac picked me up. We were on a major four-lane freeway. He was so drunk that he would bump the guardrail in the middle and then swerve across four lanes of traffic and hit the guardrail on the other side. I tried to get him to pull over, but like most drunks, he was in denial about his condition. It seemed highly likely that he was going to kill us both, so I prepared to jump.

I grabbed the keys out of the ignition, threw them in the back seat and waited for the car to slow down a bit. I opened the door just as I saw a patch of grass approaching and executed a perfect tuck and roll. Believe it or not I didn't get so much as a scratch. Did I stop hitchhiking? No.

You're probably thinking, "Geez, this girl had a death wish." You're close. I was a danger junkie. I was addicted to my own adrenaline, the Cadillac of my dysfunctions. I could produce my favorite high just by revving up my thinking. Consequently, I was always in a state of excitement. Crisis was normal for me; I knew how to cope with it. It made me feel alive when there wasn't much else in my life that made me feel at all.

After years of being a nonentity in my family, the pulse and excitement of the danger was welcome. Fear, even terror, were feelings that I had an intimate relationship with. The threat of getting harmed or killed wasn't a big deal, but the fear of being unnoticed was suffocating.

Phyllis and I arrived in Denver at Tom's house on my twentieth birthday. He met us at the door with a gun. Tom was not comfortable with fear. He slept with that gun on the nightstand and greeted every ring of the bell with it. He also was not comfortable with my coming to Denver, especially with our being homeless and jobless in his living room.

Loving me from a distance on paper and dealing with a three-dimensional woman in an intimate relationship were two very different things. Admittedly, I am not an easy person to have a relationship with. I demand that people dig deep when they are around me, and I had enough emotional baggage to fill a cargo plane at the time.

Tom retaliated the same way my father had. He waged a cold war. A week into my stay in Denver he would climb into bed and shove his back in my face, and not say a word. I was afraid of losing him and he was afraid of overtly hurting my feelings and offending my sister, whom he considered to be one of his dearest friends.

Although I eventually moved out, Tom and I continued this charade for a year and a half. I didn't have a shred of self-esteem left by the time he finally told me it was over. Many years later he apologized for the hurt he had caused me. It was evident that the guilt he had carried was every bit as heavy as the pain I had felt.

In the aftermath of this split I had plenty of offers for one-night-stands and/or romance, but it was two years before I even considered facing a relationship again.

In the meantime, I worked. I had beaten the poverty mentality, for a while anyway. I made good money slinging drinks and food. My wild personality and numerous stories and pranks were usually good for a generous tip or two. My employers loved me because I was efficient, a workaholic (yet another addiction for my collection), and would always volunteer to work the holiday shifts. I had no family around, other than Phyllis, so I dreaded holidays.

I loved waitressing and bartending. It was like being on stage all the time. I had a captive audience at each table or on every stool. Also, I was in control.

I waited on the rich and powerful on many occasions. After growing up with David, I wasn't automatically impressed by their position or their money. In my mind, power and money don't necessarily afford you the "Good Joe of the Year" award. They had to work for my respect, and I usually earned theirs.

I was waiting tables in an Irish Pub in downtown Denver, reputed to be the hub of the big boys of the oil industry. One day a party of four distinguished-looking businessmen was seated in my section. They all had on $1000 suits, but one of them was obviously "the dude" and one of them appeared to be his "yes man." The yes man seemed annoyed with me. Apparently I wasn't treating his boss with the expected servitude. He called me over and said, "Don't you know who this is?"

I responded with my usual flippant tone. "No, does he know me?"

The yes man stood up, trying to exert his nonexistent power over me. "This is Joe Blow (I don't remember the man's name), the president of Shell Oil Company."

I looked Mr. President up and down, then remarked, "That's okay, I like him anyway," and smiled. Everybody but the yes man roared. Mr. President loved it.

I have learned that very powerful and/or wealthy people are sometimes very lonely. Everybody around them kisses their ass and tells them what they think they want to hear. They are often starved for some genuine human interaction.

I pulled my best pranks on Mr. President throughout lunch, including my all-time favorite. Timing for this gag was everything. I brought out the entrees and parked them in front of each diner, while asking if I could bring anything else right away. They indicated that they were fine. I left the table and walked to the other side of the room where I could see Mr. President clearly.

As soon as I saw him put his first forkful in his mouth I came bounding up to the table, zipped his plate out from under him, and exclaimed, "Wasn't that great! Can I bring you some cheesecake for dessert?" He instinctively reached for his disappearing plate. He had his mouth full but was laughing hard, trying not to spit his food all over the table!

Mr. President wanted to fly me to his ranch in Arizona for the weekend. I declined. Probably had something to do with my aversion to letting abundance creep into my life.

Not too long after meeting the oil boys, I got a call from my father's secretary at Texaco. He was going to be in Denver on business and wanted her to schedule him some time with me.

At the time, I was tending bar in a nice, secluded place that had a fairly wealthy clientele. My father's secretary arranged for him to come see me at work for an hour. To hear him tell it later, he had come to Denver just to see me. It's amazing how he penciled in a whole week of business and golf around that one hour he had come to town to spend quality time with his daughter.

The people I was working for treated me like family and were interested in meeting the man they had heard me rant about. The day of his visit, David made a grand entrance with his driver trailing behind him. I did admire the way he commanded everybody's attention when he entered a room, like a Hollywood legend does. He didn't have to say anything. He just oozed the essence of a powerful being. I, on the other hand, was a mess. I could barely get my legs to hold me as I greeted him.

My boss, Larry, his wife, Chris, my father, his driver and I sat together at a large table. In the next hour, David found something demeaning to say about me, my job, my body and every single person in my life who wasn't present, including my sister, my mother's sister and his sister-in-law. I slumped down in my chair into a pile of non-matter while the rest of the group sat in horrified silence.

The "driver" wasn't your average chauffeur; he was another high-ranking guy in Texaco. He caught my eye a couple of times and let me know energetically that he thought my father's behavior was appalling, but apparently he was not prepared to sacrifice his working relationship with David for me.

When my hour was up, David rose, kissed me on the cheek, told me how wonderful it had been to see me and pranced to the door. I went to the kitchen and broke down. My bosses followed me in and raged about what a jerk my father had been. It was a turning point in my life. Somebody had seen him in action and validated my feelings. I wasn't crazy. This man really was emotionally battering me.

When my father returned to Texas I called my parents. I didn't have the guts to talk to "Him," so I heaped the burden on my mother. I told her that I would no longer tolerate this man in my life. I could not find peace and mental health under the weight of his judgement. Knowing that she and he were a package deal, I would have to give her up too. I also lost my brother that day; evidently he was part of the package. That made me sad, but I felt more free and alive than I had ever felt.

The one constant in my life was Phyllis. We had our moments, but all in all we coexisted very gracefully for two banged-up, bull-headed women. Of course, we were stoned, drinking or eating most of the time we were together. If we ran out of drugs or food, things got ugly.

We lived together off and on throughout our early years in Colorado, sometimes sharing a one-bedroom apartment where I had a mattress in the living room.

I usually made more money than Phyllis did because I worked for tips and she lived on a straight salary. She wasn't cut out for the service industry. She was a "Rosanne" prototype the first time she tried waiting tables. She'd dish out a lot of abuse and then rage when her victims wouldn't tip.

Because of Phyllis's rough exterior and sailor's mouth, people often didn't realize how brilliant or loving she truly was. I did. She taught me about true friendship. If you really love someone, you owe it to them to be honest, really honest.

One day, Phyllis sat me down and told me that I was behaving like my father. I was immediately pissed, but she had my attention, so I listened. She went on, "You make more money than I do. You buy groceries, pot and drinks at the bar and share them all with me. But it isn't really generous because you expect something in return. We seem to have this unspoken rule that because you have the money I'm supposed to do all the dirty work, like the dishes and the laundry and emptying the trash. If that's what you expect for your money, then you should negotiate up front. And you don't get the luxury of being the generous giver, it becomes a mutual arrangement."

Now I was really pissed, but my anger gave way to disgust. She was right – I was behaving like my father. I apologized and we changed the scope of our friendship. I started pulling my weight with the housework and shared my money because I wanted to, not because it gave me grounds to control her.

If you can't see your own behaviors clearly, you only have two chances of changing them. Either God will kick your butt, or a friend will. I had stopped listening to God, so he had sent me Phyllis. Her honesty saved me from myself more than once. She taught me well, too. I don't pull any punches with my friends, and I don't take denial for an answer. Consequently, I don't have many friends, but the ones that have hung in there with me are all I need.

Phyllis was also a fellow addict. She liked food, booze and pot as much as I did. The pot we got back then was lousy. How high you got had more to do with how much stamina and imagination you had than how much THC you actually got from the weed.

Of course, along with the pot came the munchies. Not everyone needs to smoke pot to crave junk food, but it certainly does have that effect on most people. We had a standing account at Domino's Pizza and had worn the path bare to 7-Eleven.

Phyllis's extra weight didn't seem to bother her that much. She had been much heavier when she was younger and thus was content to be the size she was. She would have liked to be lighter, but she didn't see the point of obsessing about it the way I did. No matter how many men chased me, or how many times Phyllis told me that my body was just fine, I couldn't take it in. I felt like a cow. Next to Farrah Fawcett (the barometer of acceptance in my family), I still didn't measure up.

One day after our usual binge of a large pizza and a liter of soda, I was bitching and moaning about how fat I was getting. Phyllis could take it no more. She suggested that I do what she did once in a while – stick my hand down my throat and throw up. I had never tolerated nausea or vomiting well, but on the other hand, I hadn't come to peace with my excess weight at all. I gave it a try.

Wow, what a concept! Have your cake, eat it too; get rid of it and not get fat. I was hooked! Phyllis realized right away that she had created a monster. She did it once in a while when she was uncomfortably full. I was immediately out of control. She tried to stop me but couldn't.

I was twenty-three years old. I figured that I would just do it until I could get my weight down a little and then I would get over it. Yeah, right! The biggest problem for me, with all my addictions, was that I was too smart and too functional. In my teens and early twenties I could go to work or school stoned, and still be the top achiever — except, of course, for my stint in pre-med at Austin College. I didn't smoke pot there; maybe that was the problem. (Only kidding!) Anyway, I could smoke and/or drink all night and still get where I was going alert and on time. I never gave anybody any reason to intervene in my life – except Phyllis.

Thank heavens cocaine didn't interest me. I have seen it destroy the best of people – physically, emotionally and especially financially. I just never got a buzz off it so I stuck to the cheap drugs like speed, pot, junk food, caffeine and cigarettes. Alcohol was simply for socializing. I did speed to keep from eating too much and marijuana to come down from the speed. I became what they call a "speed freak," doing it all the time. I was living on speed, cigarettes, diet soda, junk food and pot. And like most, if not all, speed freaks, I was a bitch most of the time. Speed makes you edgy because it blows your adrenal glands wide open and robs you of your sleep. Your adrenal glands are supposed to save your life if you are in danger. They can help you outrun an assailant, pick up a car if it falls on a loved one, or help you stay conscious for long periods in the wilderness for instance. Speed keeps your adrenal glands pumping all the time. Cigarettes also affect many people that way. Your body and your attitude wear out very quickly.

Phyllis told me nicely on a couple of occasions that I was doing too much speed. Like most addicts in denial, I assured her that I had everything under control. One day she'd had enough. She said, "I love you Denise, but you are no fun to be around anymore. You have a drug problem." Then she left. It hit me like a freight train.

At this point I was renting a house with a girl named Debbie, another one of those gorgeous, talented women I attracted into my life. Debbie had a beautiful figure, a pretty face, a voice like an angel and a cocaine addiction. She could have snagged any guy on the planet, but she ended up with a big, old, rough-looking biker who pimped her out for drug money.

The day Phyllis walked out on me, Debbie had a house full of guests who were all shooting-up cocaine. I locked myself in my room with my little Irish Setter puppy and cried. I stayed there for twelve hours. I decided that Phyllis was right. I was killing myself and about to lose the only person in the world that I truly cared about.

I finally came out of my room and gave away all my drugs and paraphernalia. I was going to quit drugs cold turkey. What I didn't realize at the time was that I would smoke more cigarettes, eat more and drink more. I had just rotated addictions, but it was still a step up for the time being.

I was working two jobs at the time and didn't want either of my employers to know that I had another job. I had no car, so I often had to hitchhike because the buses weren't frequent enough for my frantic schedule.

One day I was hitchhiking on Broadway, a main thoroughfare in Denver, when a nice-looking, well-dressed young guy in a new Volkswagen pulled up. I thought, "Great! At least it isn't some skuzzy bum." I hopped in and started my usual hitchhiking chatter, "So, what's your name?"

He was slow to respond. "Ahhh…John." Right then I knew I had a problem. Most people can rattle off their name without considerable thought.

"So, John, what do you do?"

"Ah…I work in this ah…rental place." Now I knew I was in trouble. My inner voice was screaming, but of course I ignored it. I needed to get where I was going and he hadn't done or said anything inappropriate yet. Yet!

We were in deep rush-hour traffic in Denver when he reached into his leather coat. I thought, "God, he's got a gun!" Instead he pulled out a switchblade, flipped it open with lightning speed and put it to my throat.

"Just do as I say and everything will be okay."

"You mean if I don't you're really going to chop me up?" I asked. He just grinned, this hideous grin. I was preparing to jump out. I figured I'd just wait until he slowed down for a light and bail out. With knife in hand, he tore my shirt and grabbed my breast. Something snapped in my brain. Now I was pissed!

I punched him square in the face. I had no training, nor had I ever really tried to hurt anyone before. I didn't hurt him, but he was so stunned that he dropped the knife and froze. I was screaming in his face a mile a minute about how sick this was and how sick he was. In a little boy's voice he murmured, "Yeah, I guess you're right."

He had stopped at a light. I opened the door and leapt out. He raced away before the light turned green, trying to get away from me as I chased him for the license plate number. I did not read the temporary plate number correctly.

The police came to my house several times. According to them a man matching an identical description had raped and killed a woman the night before just a few miles away.

Having a police detective stop by the cocaine den now and then didn't sit well with my roommate and her biker friends. They put the word out on the street that if any of them were to get arrested, they were going to gang rape me. These were the kind of guys that cops love to hassle – long hair, tattoos from head to toe and leathers. They could get arrested for jay walking. So, I packed the 1967 Plymouth that my boss had helped me buy, with my clothes and my dog and headed for Las Vegas. Change of venue time again.

FOOD FOR THOUGHT...

The legal drugs, like cigarettes and junk food, were always more dangerous for me than the illegal ones, because they are so inexpensive and accepted. It is much easier to recognize when you've done too much speed than to determine how much pizza or chocolate is a safe dose.

I now understand that a drug is a drug is a drug. It really didn't matter whether I was smoking, drinking, popping pills or eating — I was trying to get away from my pain! The pain was inside of me. Sedating it without destroying the body that hosts "me" was impossible.

My encounter with John was a mind-blower. It still didn't stop me from hitchhiking, but I did gain a healthy respect for my instincts. From then on, if something didn't feel right, I made a move, instead of ignoring my inner voice. The first time I had ignored my intuition it cost me a badly broken arm. This time I nearly got raped and killed. I guess that "sixth sense" of mine was worth listening to.

JUST FOR FUN...

As we know, speed isn't the only thing that can make women bitchy.

A minister was noting in his sermon that for every challenge or condition we might face in life, there is a Bible verse that refers to it. After the service one of his congregates approached him.

"You know, Father, I think you are mistaken. I don't believe that there are any Bible verses that mention PMS."

The stunned minister told the young woman that he would study up on it that week and have an answer for her on the following Sunday.

After the service the next week the minister approached the young woman, Bible in hand. "I found a verse pertaining to PMS," he beamed.

Holding the big Bible dramatically in his outstretched arms he read, "And Mary rode Joseph's ass all the way to Jerusalem."

An Internet jokester

"Look, Mommy, It's the Karate Lady."

The three months I spent in Las Vegas were three of the worst months of my life, possibly even worse than puberty. If you hadn't joined a labor union before rolling into town, you were pretty much screwed. I went to an employment agency I had found in the yellow pages, and without a union card, all they could offer me was a job as a stripper or a prostitute. No thanks. The sad thing was that I ended up taking as much abuse as the strippers and the working girls did but didn't get paid for it.

I believe that you get what you put out. The challenge is to change what you are putting out when you're down, so that you can change what you get back. It was clear that, during that time my energy and self-esteem were so low, I attracted every low-life on the planet to kick me.

I ended up promoting time-share condominiums for a company that was run by the mob. And I was living with the woman who was my trainer at that company. She had seven children by five different men, and beat all but one of them.

Thinking I was very tough I called the vice president of the company. I threatened to expose them because I had been cheated out of hefty commissions. So had nearly all of my co-workers.

I kid you not, they mentioned a boating trip on Lake Mead, emphasizing a pair of cement boots for me. I distinctly remember the man's secretary saying, "Little girl, you don't know who you're messing with!"

I feigned amnesia. "I don't know what you're talking about. This is all just a misunderstanding I'm sure. Well, gotta go."

The next morning I listened as Dee, the woman I was staying with, knocked her beautiful little, ten-year-old, Farrah Fawcett look-a-like daughter around. The child fled from the house and contacted the police. Dee waltzed by my door and left for work as if nothing had happened.

Dee had a record of child abuse a mile long. She had beaten her children with high-heeled shoes and curtain rods and had stabbed the oldest child in the leg with a knife. So, when the cops showed up that morning with our runaway in tow, they had no trouble believing my rendition of the events. We gathered up all the children and had a discussion, which ended in the kids deciding to leave the home.

I asked the police to give me a twenty-minute head start before they called Dee and told her that they had taken her children. Dee was one scary woman. She had mob connections too. She told me once that she was a very patient person. She could wait twenty years to seek revenge on someone.

I had already found my Irish setter a beautiful ranch to live on, so I only had a few things to throw into the Plymouth. I was on the road out of town in fifteen minutes.

I didn't make it far though. I was on the freeway, just on the outskirts of town when the car died. I tried and tried but she would not turn over. I finally started packing a bag that I could hitchhike with, resigned to leaving most of my earthly possessions behind.

I walked away from the car, about to put my thumb in the air, when I looked back at my little pile of metal and thought, "What the hell, I might as well try her one more time." She started right up. As a matter of fact, she performed so well that I got a speeding ticket upon entering Colorado. It was good to be home, I guess.

I went straight back to Phyllis. She rented me half her apartment and I found a waitressing job right away. I decided to get a life. I enrolled in night school at Arapaho Community College and signed up for a three-month course to get certified as an Emergency Medical Technician (EMT). I graduated first in my class and got a job at Reed Ambulance.

I loved my job. I had never been happier. For those of you who are ER fans, it's not like that. Once in a while you get an exciting call, but all in all you spend a lot of time polishing equipment or hauling cancer patients back and forth to chemotherapy. But if you love crisis, it's worth the wait for those life-and-death moments.

I worked with some great guys and some great patients. I learned a lot about crisis intervention and dealing with death and dying. I was quite good at ambulance work.

Leaving the service industry, though, had brought on the poverty syndrome again. I was paid ninety dollars a week to scrape people off the pavement as an ambulance attendant. I worked forty-eight hours on and forty-eight hours off, which meant I had to sleep in the station house, so I couldn't find a second job to wrap around my schedule and supplement my income. I also had to eat out or live on boxed lunches, as the ambulance house had no cooking facility.

One day we got called to a "Code Blue," meaning that the person had stopped breathing and needed resuscitating. It appeared that this old woman was quite dead when we arrived, but we didn't have the authority to make that pronouncement. My partner started chest compressions for CPR and I reached for the Ambu-bag, a cup that fits over the patient's mouth and nose, with an attached bag you squeeze to force air into the their lungs. The Ambu-bag malfunctioned, so I had to begin mouth-to-mouth resuscitation.

Shortly thereafter, the contents of this old, drunk, dead woman's stomach came up into my mouth. I gagged, cleaned us up and resumed mouth-to-mouth until the fire department arrived and called the time of death. I was pissed!

When we got back to the station I was bitching pretty loudly about the Ambu-bag, still traumatized from swapping stomach contents with a dead person. My complaint did not fall on sympathetic ears. I was fired on the spot. No room for discussion, just "Get the hell out!" I walked the five miles home in a daze, trying to figure out what had just happened. I cried most of the way.

The walk did me good though. By the time I had reached the apartment, I had a plan. I would go back to school and get a nursing license. Nurses have the most clout in the emergency medical field, other than doctors, who rarely leave the hospitals. I wanted to work on the flight-for-life choppers. More education would be good.

I got yet another waitressing job and enrolled in nursing school, once again at Arapaho Community College. Before long I had three jobs and a full class load, but I loved school and excelled in all my studies.

I was now involved with a guy named Vern who was taking Kung Fu lessons. He lived for karate. I had the opportunity to take Tae Kwon-Do for a P.E. credit. I thought it would help me lose a few pounds, get in shape and have something to share with my new boyfriend.

I was in terrible shape, could barely run a block or two, smoked cigarettes and pot, drank alcohol and ate junk. I had been a vegetarian for five years at this point, but that didn't mean that I knew a darn thing about healthy eating. I had just eliminated meat products from my diet. And, I was still bulimic.

I remember my first day of Tae Kwon-Do as if it were yesterday. The advanced students were all decked out in white uniforms with colored belts, and we starry-eyed beginners were assembled on the other side of the gym. When the instructor entered the room, a strange feeling washed over me. It was similar to the séance incident, a "knowing" and a "vision" that came to me.

The instructor was a tiny Korean man named Yung Chul Ra, a sixth degree black-belt instructor who had a charismatic smile and spoke very little English. He was also missing his right hand, but he hid it very well.

At the time he was happily in love with a little redheaded woman named Mary. But the moment I set eyes on Yung Chul Ra, I knew that we would be lovers someday and I knew that I would excel past the level of any student he'd ever trained. I had no sound reason to believe all that, but I knew it as sure as I knew my name.

Tae Kwon-Do became the most powerful, driving addiction in my life. I excelled at it because it gave me an outlet for the mountain of rage I was harboring. I got to scream and kick at things and be aggressive. Even given the terrible shape I was in, Yung could see that I was special.

My car had long since died and I was back to buses and hitchhiking. (Spirit apparently wants me outside, walking.) I would hitchhike all over Denver to attend the various classes that Yung taught. Many times I would end up at Denver University at night to work out in his final class before he returned to his private school in Longmont where he lived, thirty miles away.

Oftentimes Mr. Ra would give me a ride home or to the bus. He deeply admired my dedication and commitment. No other beginner trained more than three classes a week. I was sometimes attending three a day. He also recognized that I had been very abused in my life, as he had, and that Tae Kwon-Do was a ticket to freedom for me, as it had been for him.

Yung also valued my friendship. Everybody in his life treated him like some monk or guru who was unapproachable. He needed a friend who would treat him as an equal, and he needed someone who would correct his English and teach him more. I became that friend.

At five-foot-five, Yung was small even for a Korean. His father had left the family when he was very young, so he had been raised by a house-full of women. At sixteen he lost his right hand and forearm while working in a factory. He caught it in a machine. He endured many months in a crude Korean hospital, an experience, which scared him away from the medical profession for life.

As a small, handicapped, Korean teen he was battered, bullied, and abused by other teens. Hands are considered sacred in the Orient; losing one was a disgrace for him. He went to the local Tae Kwon-Do hall for refuge. He washed the feet of the instructor, cleaned the gym, and helped teach in return for lessons. He slept on a cement floor and shared a blanket with two other students, Jhoon Ree and Nam Te Hi, who also went on to be among the top Tae Kwon-Do Masters in the world.

Their master, General Choi Hong Hi, had developed Tae Kwon-Do for the Korean army while sitting in a Japanese prisoner of war camp during World War II. Yung literally got it from the horse's mouth.

Mr. Ra had taught Tae Kwon-Do and performed demonstrations around the world before being brought to the United States by our government to train servicemen. God walked me into his humble classroom in an obscure community college and changed my life forever. I was ripe for change, as things at home were not good.

Vern had lost his job in an electrical supply company and had slid into a deep depression because he couldn't find work. One day I picked up an application that he had filled out to see if there was some advice I could give him. I was floored. The man was illiterate. He did not even know that the first word of a sentence is capitalized and that you need a period at the end. Nor could he write or spell. It was no wonder he couldn't find work. I had lived with him for over a year and hadn't had a clue. His depression was getting so deep that I could barely reach him.

Meanwhile, Mary had thrown Yung out and he was quite depressed and angry. Not one to let the two most important men in my life suffer alone, I started a nervous breakdown. I hadn't realized how much stress I had been feeling trying to juggle these two men, their emotional baggage, my own issues, a full class load and three part-time jobs. Every other waking moment I was obsessed with Tae Kwon-Do.

I was sitting in our apartment one day when a rush of emotions came over me. I reached for a joint, then of course some sweets. Neither of those sedated the pain this time. I felt I was going to explode if I didn't get some help.

I curled up in a ball and cried for hours. I was totally out of control. I had very little money so I couldn't imagine there was any help out there I could afford, but a little voice said, "Get on the phone. You'll never know what you can get unless you try."

I called the county mental health center. They agreed to see me right away on a sliding scale. I began therapy for three dollars a week. Perhaps there was a God. I felt a glimmer of hope.

I was more a robot than a person for the next few months. In order to hold it together in school and at work,

I had to shut down my emotions after therapy. I felt like a machine with an on-off switch.

I was nearing the end of my first year of nursing school, so I quit two of my jobs and distributed my time among Tae Kwon-Do, Yung, Vern and therapy. I was now seeing the therapist twice a week. Yung and I were spending more time together outside of class and Vern was getting much harder to handle as he sank deeper and deeper into depression.

One day Vern and I were having dinner with the couple that lived in the apartment below us. Robin was a very large woman. She was my first true study in the subject of denial. She weighed a good three hundred pounds but would say things like, "Gosh, I feel bloated today. If I could just lose these last fifteen pounds..." She got annoyed when she was pregnant and nobody noticed or commented. (Like you're going to risk approaching an obese woman and saying, "Gee, when's the baby due?") This particular day however, it was a blessing that she was the size she was.

We were all drinking wine. Vern had done some speed also. He was talking about the Samurai warriors and how they would slice their bellies open. He appeared to be in some sort of trance and was gesturing as he spoke as if he were pulling a knife across his midriff. Understand: Vern was a good-sized guy. He was about six-foot-two, lifted weights and worked out constantly.

A few minutes later, I was sitting in the living room chatting with Robin's husband when there was a commotion in the kitchen. Apparently, Robin had tackled Vern because he had gotten out one of her butcher knives and was about to filet himself open. Robin wrestled the knife away from him, but he got away from all of us and ran out to the parking lot.

He began beating up cars with his bare fists, bashing in the hoods and windshields. I was trying to talk him down when he turned on me. He was screaming at me and threatening to kill me. I called the police. They took him away.

They released him to me the next day. The man they gave me, though, was a broken human being. He had recently revealed to me that he had been molested at eight by one of his mother's closest male friends. He had never told another living soul about the sexual assault. It was eating him alive.

I stayed with Vern for another six months out of guilt. During that time, I also started an affair with one of my professors who told me years later that he was emotionally devastated when I broke it off. I carried the guilt of abandoning those two men for many years.

One night Vern lost it on me again. By then we were living in a trailer. I packed up my things about midnight, hid them under the trailer and took off with my sleeping bag. I couldn't keep living this way. I didn't love him anymore and I couldn't help him.

I slept by the railroad tracks most of the night before moving to a park. I had a knife in one hand, my fighting sticks in the other and one eye open. I moved every couple of hours to keep from being cased by potential assailants. Phyllis wasn't around or reachable so, after two sleepless nights, I called Yung. He came and got me and brought me to his Longmont gym. All my belongings had been stolen from under the trailer while I had been dodging boogiemen in the park. I was down to the shirt on my back.

Yung had just opened a second gym in Loveland, Colorado, which was about sixty miles north of Denver. He commuted between Loveland, Longmont, Denver and Lakewood (west of Denver) to teach, a total of 180 miles some days.

He told me that I could move into his Loveland gym, with a few conditions. I had to give up drugs, alcohol and cigarettes cold turkey, and I had to tell all my friends that I was moving back East. He wanted me to make a clean break from my toxic lifestyle. I agreed, quit my last job, and dropped out of nursing school. Yung arrogantly predicted that I wouldn't last a week.

I had a mattress in the men's dressing room to sleep on, which I propped up against the wall during the day. I had a skillet to cook in and I either bathed in the Longmont gym when we were there, or in Lake Loveland. We only had a sink and a toilet in the Loveland gym.

I had reached the level of blue belt by now. Blue belt represents about a year's worth of training, which is usually enough to make you cocky, stupid and dangerous to yourself. I trained or helped teach anywhere from three to eight hours a day. My fellow students trained three to four times a week.

Yung also got me up at 4 a.m. to run six miles every morning. Eventually we ran eight. In the afternoons I would practice my patterns and kick at the bag before opening the gym for evening classes. I traveled all over with Yung and I was truly in heaven. For the first time in my life I was dedicated to not screwing it up.

As I knew we would, Yung and I became lovers. It was a bumpy beginning, however. He was still in love with Mary. I was still reeling from the guilt of Vern, and emotionally attached to the professor I had let go of. But our friendship flourished and so did I as a student.

Yung drove me harder than any other student he had. I got angry with him one day for being so mean to me. He lovingly explained that if he didn't love me he wouldn't waste his time pushing me so hard. He was teaching me the best of what he knew and expected me to give 100 percent. From that day on I was like a sponge. If he could dish it out, I could take it.

I outlasted his prediction by ten years. I lived in one Do-Jang (the Korean term for training hall) or another with Yung for five years. Then, with his blessings, I opened my own school in Loveland after he had closed his.

I earned a third degree black belt, was the only woman allowed to compete in the men's advanced black-belt division, and won my share of competitions. I maintained a school full of talented, loving, and giving men, women and children and found some peace in my life. I also acquired an exercise disorder to accompany my other dysfunctions.

I had quit smoking pot and cigarettes. Once in a great while I would share a joint with someone I trusted not to destroy my life and my reputation, but I was no longer addicted. I had a beer now and then with my students after testings or competitions, but didn't care much for alcohol anymore. I couldn't however, break my sugar addiction, or consequently, the bulimia.

I also went some rounds with anorexia. It was like a switch that turned on and off in my mind. Normally I couldn't stop eating, but once in a while I just couldn't get myself to put food in my mouth. I would run, train, and teach for days on end without eating a single scrap. I knew I needed to eat but food seemed like the enemy. That damned Farrah Fawcett thing kept swimming in my head.

I so desperately wanted to be thinner. Even though I was only about ten pounds over my ideal weight, I was solid muscle, which is even harder to take off. That perfect size-four body was still out of reach, especially since I have size eight bones at best.

I believe that there were a few people in my life along the way who suspected that I was bulimic, but none dared confront me on it, except one — Yung. He did say one day that he suspected I vomited my food. I lied. I was too ashamed to tell him the truth. I wish I had. I know he would have stood by and helped me.

I couldn't stop overtraining either, even when it was obvious that my body needed a rest. After breaking a bone, I'd come back from the hospital and go straight to the gym to practice. In 1987 I was covered in plaster most of the year. I broke my right hand in January punching boards, my left hand in February teaching a rape prevention class and a bone in my neck in April just spinning to kick. Granted, I did a lot of dangerous things, but I would not have sustained as many injuries if I had not been abusing my body so hard with junk food, bulimia and overtraining.

I love to break boards. I would face a huge pile of them fearlessly. Putting my foot through a three-inch stack of pine (four three-quarter-inch pieces held together) was the most satisfying rush of power I had ever experienced, even more exhilarating than jumping out of a plane.

I could out-break the guys because I trained so much more. Breaking is about speed, focus and mind power, not size or brawn. Yung used to say, "Some ladies you give to flowers; Denise, she love breaking board so much."

My body began to seriously deteriorate from malnutrition and excessive exercise. Some days I hurt so badly that I could hardly walk. I had three doctors tell me that I was going to end up in a wheelchair if I didn't quit Tae Kwon-Do. But I would have died before giving it up; it was my life.

For the year prior to my second degree black-belt testing I had to quit kicking with my right leg. Each of us has a dominant leg, just as we are either right-handed or left-handed. I had to do all my board breaking for second degree with my nondominant leg because of the damage I had done to my right hip. It was ludicrous to be training at all, but it did cause me to become ambidextrous.

I finally found a chiropractor who could see that I wasn't going to stop, so he set out to teach me how to take better care of my body. Dr. Kerry Randa became one of my dearest friends. He is the only reason that I am not in a wheelchair. If I could have told him about my eating disorder, he could have helped me with that as well. But I couldn't tell anyone.

Kerry accompanied me to the Olympic trials in Dayton, Ohio, for the 1988 Olympic Games. Although Tae Kwon-Do was only slated to be an Olympic demonstration sport in Korea, I still had to compete to make the team. I had been training with the Olympic trainers in Colorado Springs and had made it to the nationals.

In the final moments of the last round of the last match I had to compete in to make the Olympic team, I spun to throw a hook kick and snapped my foot. I had been training so hard that my bone just fractured from the stress of my spinning on it. I never finished the round. I might not have won anyway. I'll never know. For me it was a tragic and emotional experience. But Paula had flown out to support me and Kerry was a rock, as always. Their validation had made it worth the trip.

In addition, I was extremely unhappy with the way the trials were being handled. Integrity, respect and manners were secondary to winning for most of the competitors. That didn't sit well with me. Yung had instilled much higher values than that in all his students. But, then, he had never wanted me to go in the first place.

Tae Kwon-Do was a spiritual endeavor to him. It wasn't about winning or losing. The only reason that he ever hosted tournaments at all was that he would have gone out of business if he hadn't. Americans love those trophies and ribbons. By the time I hit third degree blackbelt, I saw and felt what Yung had felt. Tae Kwon-Do is a path to peace, empowerment and enlightenment, not a violent or competitive sport.

Returning to my gym from lunch one day, wearing my uniform pants and a T-shirt as usual, I spotted a little boy and his mother walking down the sidewalk across the street. The boy pointed excitedly and exclaimed, "Look, Mommy, it's the Karate Lady!"

I was somebody. I had a life!

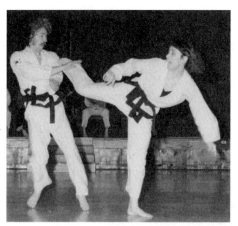

Sparring at my second degree blackbelt testing with Gary Thompson.

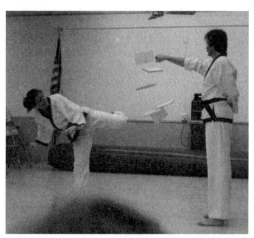

Three-board, suspended, hook-kick break.

FOOD FOR THOUGHT...

I did a few spots on TV, had some nice articles written about me and was invited to show off my students at local fairs and openings. It was a great life. Most of all, I treasure the friends I made and the wisdom and maturity I gained in that very special decade of my existence.

I could write a whole book on my Tae Kwon-Do career.

I came out the other side a very different person. I had gained personal power, the respect of my students and my peers, and a presence that had peeled the "Abuse Me" sign off my back. Imagine what walking into a room and having seventy men, women and children snap to attention and bow with respect means to a person who had been totally powerless in childhood!

Now when I walk down the sidewalk, I exude a totally different energy. Safety and personal power come from within. It isn't my skills that make me safe. It is the self-confidence I have gained.

I look back on my career as a full-time athlete and wonder what I would have accomplished if I had known then what I know now about food. I could have been world-class if I hadn't been malnourished. I had all the other ingredients it takes. And I watch so many fine athletes totally ignoring the fact that what you put in this very sophisticated machine makes a difference in its performance. What a shame!

JUST FOR FUN...

Yung (who later earned his citizenship and proudly changed his name to Daniel) loved to learn new English phrases. One of my favorites was "piece of cake."

One day he asked, "What's this mean?" I explained it to him to the best of my ability.

Soon after, Daniel saw an opportunity to use the new phrase he had learned in a conversation. He carefully led up to the punchline and then beamed as he spouted, "Piece of chalk-ret!" "Chalk-ret" was his pronunciation for "chocolate."

I explained to him that I didn't know why, but it had to be cake.

At the next opportunity, he excitedly tried again, "Piece of chalk-ret cake!"

VINCE

During my Tae Kwon-Do career, a couple of other people touched me so profoundly that I am going to afford them each a chapter. First Vince.

One sunny afternoon, about six months after I had moved into the Loveland gym, Vince Stephens came bouncing through the door. I was twenty-five years old at the time, a full-time athlete and a year and a half into my bulimia.

Vince always had that "cat that swallowed the canary" air about him. He introduced himself and began his sales pitch for the minitrampoline he was trying to sell me. I thanked him but assured him that the trampoline would not have much advantage for me as I already trained hard for four to eight hours a day. That opened the door for Vince's other sales pitch. He wanted to sell me some vitamins.

I was about to give him the bum's rush when he started to unfold his life story. I might have a few of the details wrong but this is the story he told me — and Phil Donahue's audience after hitting the talk show trail. He also wrote a small book that was on the market for a while. I haven't been able to find him or the book in the past ten years. Where are you, Vince?

Vince had played bass guitar in a band as a young adult. At some point he had begun to notice that his dexterity wasn't what it used to be. He also had begun to have problems with other motor skills, as well as his speech. After much poking and prodding and many endless tests, Vince was diagnosed with multiple sclerosis.

I don't remember how many years he said it took him to fall into the abyss — I think eight — but he ended up on his deathbed. He no longer had the use of his arms or legs, and he couldn't feed himself or hold up his head. Eventually he couldn't even speak.

The finest doctors in the country, including those at the famed Mayo Clinic, could not help him. They said that the best they could do was keep him comfortable with large doses of morphine until he died.

With the help of his devoted wife, Shirley, he wrote to doctors all over the world. A few wrote back and said that they were beginning to believe that M.S. was a nutritional disease and that he should go on a macrobiotic diet and take mass doses of supplements. I believe some of the physicians who responded even offered Vince some recommendations on which combinations of vitamins and minerals to try. I specifically remember that he took high doses of organic alfalfa tablets.

As I recall, he said it took him two years to ascend from quadriplegia to a wheelchair and two more years after that before he was up and dancing and talking to Phil. The man who bounced into our gym that day showed no signs of ever having missed a beat in life. He was so healthy and vibrant that I might not have believed him were it not for the numerous newspaper clippings he showed me as our friendship progressed.

His wife had an amazing story to tell as well. Shirley's family was struggling with arthritis. One of her relatives, her sister I think, had been a concert pianist before succumbing to crippling arthritis in her hands. Shirley's hands had also become painfully crippled with arthritis.

While helping Vince with his recovery she decided to see what she could do for her own ailment. She adhered to the strict diet that Vince was on, although perhaps not quite as rigidly, and she, too, took mass doses of organic alfalfa. She started with sixty tablets a day and backed down to twenty after beating her arthritis. That's right, she beat it all together. Racehorses are fed alfalfa; dogs and cats eat grass when they get sick. It made sense to me.

What I have learned since meeting Shirley suggests that arthritis is basically about toxic joints. The body is not detoxifying efficiently and it is depositing waste in the joints.

What didn't make sense to me was that the former concert pianist would not listen to her. Even with Shirley standing in her living room, saying, "Look at me, my arthritis is gone," her sister had apparently insisted, "That's impossible. That can't work." A concert pianist who couldn't even play "Chopsticks" anymore — you'd think she would have tried anything! I can see being afraid to try Ritalin or morphine, but alfalfa is just animal fodder, like grass.

Hearing this story planted the first seed in my head that dis-ease, for some people, is a choice. This woman was refusing to try a natural remedy with which someone she loved had experienced miraculous results. Having Vince and Shirley in my life was to be my second exposure to the phenomenon of denial. They were surrounded by it.

Vince was deeply dedicated to helping other M.S. sufferers. Besides writing a book and speaking nationally on the subject, he pioneered an intense local effort. He met with insurance companies and cut deals with the folks at Meals on Wheels. He arranged to have the macrobiotic foods and organic supplements paid for and delivered directly to the homes of the M.S. patients he had found in the area.

To his utter amazement, most of them wouldn't even try the foods or supplements, although Vince was standing in the room with documentation to prove his success on the regime. Did they not want to get well? Were their cookies and hamburgers more important than their legs or their speech? Vince didn't get it. Neither did I at the time. Eventually, Vince became very bitter and gave up trying to help other people with multiple sclerosis.

Vince did not stick to as severe a diet after he regained his health as he had on the road to recovery, but he was very careful about one thing — sugar. Vince said that even one doughnut would make his hands start shaking again. He also said that he hadn't cured his M.S., he had just learned to control it. It became a lifetime arrangement with his body: "I'll do right by you, and you do right by me."

If the concept that disease can be a choice is new to you, then I would highly recommend that you pick up any of Louise Hay's books. Louise Hay believes that there are underlying emotions that we may be unaware of, or afraid to look at, that lead us into physical illness. Louise has many fabulous books on the market that can assist us in our recovery. My personal nightstand favorite is You Can Heal Your Life, from her publishing company, Hay House.

Shortly after meeting Vince I became very ill. I went from being able to train eight hours a day to throwing a few kicks and seeing stars and having to sit down. I went for some blood tests, and when the results came in the doctor called me at the gym and remarked, "Your blood count is so low I can't believe you're still walking around."

He wanted me to come in for some medications. Instead, I called Vince.

I bought a multivitamin supplement, some iron and some protein powder. Not only did I get my strength and stamina back, but for the first time, I discovered that exercise doesn't have to be painful. I could run six or eight miles and enjoy every step instead of just persevering through the torture. I could jump up and kick for an hour without my face turning beet red and my heart trying to leap out of my chest. Who knew?

I finally talked Yung into trying some of the supplements, but they had no effect on him. He ate whole foods and trained in a healthy way, so he wasn't depleted or suffering in the first place.

I would have died from my bulimia years ago if I hadn't learned how to give my body back some of the vitamins and minerals my bulimia robbed it of by supplementing with vitamins. Supplements are helpful on the road to rejuvenating yourself, but ultimately one must stop consuming toxins and find whole, energized foods to fuel their body, not little magic bullets. That's why they're called supplements!

Unfortunately, in spite of meeting Vince and learning how harmful sugar is, I couldn't break my addiction to it. In time I became critically ill. It wasn't the first time, nor would it be the last.

I need to back up and give you a little history. My medical problems began just after I'd moved to Denver at nineteen. I had not yet developed my eating disorder or become an athlete, but I had experienced some serious health problems.

I would be walking along in a department store or at work and have a shooting pain up my rectum that would drop me to the floor. I had test after test until the doctors had exhausted all my money. All they could say was "You have a spastic colon or something. Perhaps it's a virus.

We could run some more tests." I gave up and lived with the pain.

A year or two later I got a bad case of salmonella (food poisoning for those of you who haven't had the pleasure). I was really sick with horrible vomiting, severe diarrhea, and terrible stomach pains. This occurred shortly after I had begun my friendship with Yung. He came to my apartment that Friday and I asked him to take me to the hospital, but he refused. I didn't realize at the time that he was afraid the doctors might kill me, based on his own devastating experience in a Korean hospital as a teen.

Instead, he sat by my bed all weekend and told me to meditate. When he finally left on Sunday night, I hitchhiked to Swedish Hospital. There they told me that I was so dehydrated I was in danger of having a heart attack, but that I had to leave because they were a private hospital and I had no insurance. I hitchhiked further across Denver to Colorado General Hospital, hunched over in pain. They treated me for salmonella.

I never really got well, though, and simply added abdominal pains to my list of symptoms. I had a battery of tests. They were beginning to believe that I had endometriosis. Endometriosis is a condition in which some of the tissue of the uterine lining that produces blood and sheds every month somehow gets outside of the uterus. Those cells still do their thing each month with the rise and fall of the hormones, sometimes causing excessive internal bleeding and pain.

I had a laparoscopy, a procedure where they cut a little hole in my belly button and a little hole down by my pubis, then blew me up with gas and peeked inside. They found nothing.

Yung was scared to death, but he came to the hospital and waited for me to return from surgery. He held my hand as my body convulsed and I puked green for hours from the general anesthetic. It did nothing to ease his distrust of doctors, or mine.

After I got through puking they decided they should do a biopsy for Hodgkin's disease. The surgeon who had done the laparoscopy said to me, "Darn, we could have done that while we had you under." He thought that they had already performed a biopsy on me and was quite annoyed that they had ordered the laparascopy first.

You might be thinking, "Well, if you had told the doctors about your eating disorder, they could have diagnosed you." I did bring up the subject of diet. I was prepared to tell them if I thought it would help them save me. Before I got very far in the discussion about diet, the head of the cancer unit for Colorado General Hospital — reputed to be one of the best cancer treatment centers in the world — told me that diet had nothing to do with the fact that I might have cancer. So I couldn't see the point in telling them about my destructive eating habits.

I knew he was wrong, though. How could food not have something to do with health? You can't put milk in your gas tank and expect high performance from your car. You have to give it the right fuel. And our bodies are certainly more sophisticated and sensitive than an automobile.

They scheduled the biopsy for a week or so later. I was awake for the surgery, which should have been a simple outpatient procedure. After I was given a local anesthetic on my neck, the surgeon was to take out a small piece of tissue to send to the lab.

The surgeon must have been a chain-smoker for his smoke-laden breath gagged me throughout the surgery, as he wheezed and coughed a few inches from my face. He literally sawed on my neck as though it were a piece of leather, then bandaged me up and sent me home.

A few hours later, I could barely breathe. I had one of my students take me to the emergency room. I was admitted to the hospital. Apparently I had complications thanks to Dr. Marlboro Hacksaw who had performed my biopsy. My throat was swelling shut. They wanted to make sure I made it through the night, all at my expense, of course. (Yes, I'm bitter towards the medical profession. But I realize that they do save many lives. I can only imagine, though, the good they could do if they would get educated about food and educate their patients!) I was released in a few days, still waiting for the results of the test to come back.

Paula flew out from the East Coast to be with me throughout this ordeal. It was a tense week for me and Paula. The burden of being my surrogate mother was wearing her down. I owe Paula a lot for the twenty years she had been my only family, but this particular day she wasn't such a wonderful friend.

I remember standing at the sink washing dishes, with this monster bandage on my throat. We had run out of polite conversation to fill up the hours while nervously waiting for the test results.

Suddenly, she blurted out, "It's not fair that you don't have insurance. If you die, I'll have to pay to bury you." I'm sure if she could have taken it back after it fell out of her mouth, she would have. We exchanged a few words before I told her to get out.

Before leaving the next morning, she left me a check for $500 with a nice note saying it was a donation to the "Send Denise to the Olympics" fund. She has apologized more times than is necessary for that remark over the years. I have long since forgiven her; I hope she has let herself off the hook.

The results of my biopsy came back negative. The doctor admitted that they didn't know what I was suffering from, that it was probably one of some two thousand known viruses. They could run some more tests. I said, "No thanks."

I sought out a little old man named Dr. Ballman, an acupuncturist. Doc Ballman had trained in China and developed an amazing gift for diagnosis, for a white guy. I told him nothing about my symptoms. He ran his hand down my thigh and said, "Seems like salmonella." I wondered if the salmonella had stayed in my system all these years and had been eating away at my organs one at a time.

I received two weeks of acupuncture treatments from Doc. He also gave me some Pau D'Arco tea and some barley green (more grass). Along with that I decided that I would do what Vince had done. I got a few books on macrobiotics and began hunting down herbs and exotic roots and such. In a month I was pain-free. It was also the first month in four years that I hadn't vomited my food.

Of course, though, as soon as I felt better I returned to my old favorite toxic foods and my eating disorder came right back to haunt me. Only now I was very careful to keep up the supplements. It was to be another ten years of "patch and tape," as my mother would say, before my body gave out again.

While we are on the subject of Vince and Shirley, there is another facet of my martial arts career that I must tell you about.

Shortly after I earned my first degree black-belt, I was approached by a friend of mine. She was a member of the Sexual Assault Advocacy Team in Loveland. These women went through crisis intervention training and volunteered their time to help women who had been raped.

They would meet the victim at the hospital and support her emotionally as she went through the difficult task of being examined physically and questioned by the hospital staff and the police. They would sometimes even accompany the survivor into court for the trial in the unlikely event of an arrest and prosecution of the assailant.

These advocates were not in denial about the horrors of sexual assault and wanted to learn some techniques to make themselves and their families safer.

I set out to develop a program that drew from my personal experiences on the streets and included some street-fighting techniques I developed with Yung's help. It took most people years to become a seasoned street fighter by working their way through the ranks of Tae Kwon-Do. I needed to teach these women something in a few hours.

Shirley Stevens was in one of my very first rape prevention programs. One night I was teaching my students a technique for releasing someone who had grabbed them by the wrist. There was one technique for a mildly annoying assailant — say a bar drunk — and one technique for a more serious situation, such as someone trying to haul them off to a bush or van.

They were very effective techniques and the ladies had them down in no time, Shirley being one of the best. As she tells it, she went home that night to Vince who was very curious to hear about what she had learned. He egged her on with some cocky rap — "I'm a man and you're a woman, you can't handle me."

Shirley didn't bat a pretty little eye. She said, "Okay, grab my wrist." Bye-bye Vince. Shirley laid him out cold in the living room. The next time I saw Vince he had apparently coughed up that canary and swallowed a little crow instead.

Vince will always be a hero to me, though. Facing our emotions and addictions is the most grueling work there is. It takes a lot of courage!

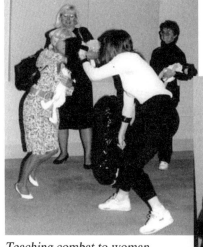

Teaching combat to woman carrying purses and babies, and wearing high heels.

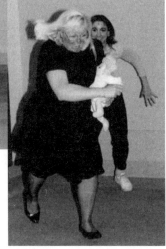

Jan Clemons from St. Mary's Women's Center – an angel on the run.

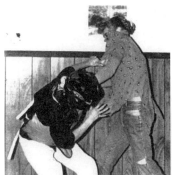

That's me in the white pants getting the crap beat out of me.

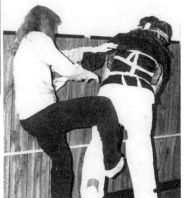

Ouch! I trained them too well.

FOOD FOR THOUGHT...

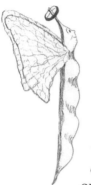

Meeting Vince profoundly changed my life. It took me a long time after he educated me about food to actually turn my destructive eating habits around. But if I had not met Vince, I would probably be dead.

Seeing that Vince had recovered from the later stages of a very debilitating disease gave me hope. I finally believed that I could beat my bulimia and undo the damage I had done to myself with this ugly disease. Without that hope, I might not have found the courage to face the long road ahead to recovery. Thanks, Vince!

As for the denial thing, I continued to study the phenomenon in others, which eventually helped me break through my own denials.

JUST FOR FUN...

The essence of what I taught in my "Street Savvy" classes was how to exude that "Don't mess with me, I can take care of myself" energy, whether the person could follow through or not. This is a cute story about the power of living that philosophy.

During the stage when I was a cocky, dangerous-to-myself blue belt, I was walking down a residential street in Denver about two one afternoon. I began to pass a house that had a flimsy, thigh-high fence around it and a very vicious Doberman Pinscher pup in the yard. As soon as he spotted me, he went berserk.

In seconds he stepped over the fence as if it weren't there. That brought us nose to nose. He was barking, growling and showing off his teeth; I was in fighting stance, trying to figure out what the hell to do.

I decided to throw a kick in front of his nose and see if I could get him to back off. I succeeded in throwing a very nice front kick, which landed a half-inch from his nose. He backed up for a second, took a puzzled glance at me then came right back barking and snarling. I tried again. I threw another perfect kick at his nose. He backed up a little farther and pondered a little longer, then came right back into the fight.

By this time I was getting really nervous. I wasn't sure that I knew how to stop this dog. Elbows and feet are very different from teeth and claws. I chose to kick at his nose one more time.

Bam! It snapped mere millimeters from his snout. He slid back, thought hard for a moment, then jumped the fence, sped across the lawn, jumped the fence on the other side of the property and took off, never looking back.

I collected myself and walked to the nearest pay phone. I called the local animal control agency and told them that this vicious dog was out running around, noting that it was time for the kids to get out of school. They told me they would send the dogcatcher immediately. He would pick me up and I could show him where I had encountered the dog.

As we were headed back in the doggy paddy wagon to the house where the dog had been, I was telling the dogcatcher about Kung-Fu fighting with the Doberman. His attitude was "Yeah, sure lady, whatever." He was laughing at me.

When we pulled up to the house the dog was standing in the front yard once again. The dogcatcher got out and told me to stay in the truck. He carefully approached the yard, but as soon as he opened the front gate, the dog went ballistic again. The Doberman stood on his hind legs, and planted his front paws on the man's chest, preparing to rip his face off.

I got out of the truck. I didn't know what I was going to do, but felt I had to make a move to help the guy. As I walked through the front gate, the dog turned and looked at me. Without hesitation he took off running, jumped the fence and was gone.

The dogcatcher was flabbergasted! I could see him trying to register what had just happened: "That dog's afraid of her?!!" Without saying a word, he drove me back to where he had picked me up. I quietly gloated the whole way.

LOWELL

Lowell is another person who graced my life in a way that merits a chapter of his own. Actually, Lowell was such a major player in my evolution that he deserves two chapters in my life story.

Yung (excuse me, it's Daniel now) and I had ended our romance but were to remain close friends. He will always have a place in my heart and my respect. I know he feels the same about me.

After Daniel, I had been through another relationship with a wonderful man who was raising his young daughter on his own. I owe Jim and Chrissy a lot. I was not the wife-and-mother type, however, and when I pointed that out to Jim, he agreed. It was time to go our separate ways. It was painful for all of us, but a wise decision.

I mention Jim because I think that it is interesting that as soon as I let go of the relationship with Jim, Lowell appeared in my life. I walked away from Jim because I wasn't cut out to be a mother, and then, well you'll see.

By the time I met Lowell I was twenty-eight, a second-degree black-belt and living in my own Tae Kwon-Do studio in Loveland, Colorado. It was a 3000-square-foot building that had been a bar before we remodeled it. I slept in the back in what had been a beer cooler. I had a living room (work-out space) that you could land a plane in and a spacious office full of plants. I loved this place.

Many nights I would dim the lights, put on some music, and spend all night practicing slow motion techniques or kicks on the bag. It was truly nirvana! If I hadn't had this interval of peace in my life, and if I hadn't acquired some maturity by then, I would never have been able to handle Lowell.

I was working out one afternoon when a woman brought a young boy to my gym. She said that he, her son Lowell, was being beaten up at school and harassed because of the behaviors his autism generated. The school counselor had suggested that she bring him to me. A number of children who were acting out at school, or too shy to fit in, had blossomed in my classes.

I can't take all the credit, however. I had many special black-belt and lower-belt students who helped me with the kids. Mike Lasner was the best of the pack. This man had an endless supply of love and patience. Thank God, because I didn't when Lowell came into my life.

Lowell was ten years old at the time, a sweet-looking kid, very slight, with big eyes and a magical smile, always in perpetual motion. I knew next to nothing about autism when I agreed to take on Lowell. I thought it was about children who lived in their own silent world and couldn't communicate or be reached.

That is sometimes the case, but not always. Autism, I was to find out, is an umbrella word that covers a lot of different behaviors. Autism is described as a neurological disorder that most greatly affects the senses. Lowell could not process all the sounds and sights and feelings that his body received, so he was constantly overwhelmed by the outside world.

Imagine that you have the record player blaring, the TV going, somebody talking to you, a person holding each hand and a psychedelic light show going on. Autism is something like that – every moment of the day.

Lowell would get into what I call loops, focusing on the same question or topic for months — or even years — on end. He was the consummate "Rainman," that wonderful character Dustin Hoffman played in the award-winning movie of the same name about an autistic man. Fortunately, K-Mart wasn't Lowell's subject of choice, like Rainman. But six months of the same question about waterfalls could make me buggy as well.

He would ask me the same question three times in the space of five minutes. If I said, "Well, what do you think?" he could rattle off a very eloquent answer — but he couldn't stop himself from asking the question again in thirty seconds. I asked him on a few occasions why he was asking me a question that I had just answered. He became very upset and said, "I don't know." He simply couldn't control his brain.

Lowell was part of the general population of my school for only a few months. One day I was trying to teach a full class of dedicated martial artists while rocking Lowell in my arms as he spouted obscenities at the top of his lungs. I realized this wasn't fair to the rest of the students, so I started giving Lowell private lessons.

Lowell was bright enough to learn some basic techniques but he really wasn't interested. What he needed most was some personal power and a friend. Before long we gave up on the lessons and just spent time together.

Lowell was an expensive habit for me. We could blow through sixty bucks in an afternoon playing pinball or video games, traveling to Denver for some fun or eating out. But if they had a "Lowell University of Life" and charged a $100,000 for tuition, it would be money well spent. The following is a collection of my favorite Lowell stories, in no particular order.

Lowell and I traveled all over Colorado and occasionally Wyoming. He enjoyed my old Volvo, in which we spent many quality hours. When I couldn't handle his constant chatter anymore, I would tell Lowell that I needed to concentrate on my driving. That would slow him down for a minute or two.

One day we decided to head for Elitches, the amusement park in Denver. It was about an hour's drive so I was pretty well stark raving mad by the time we arrived there. My plan was to keep Lowell busy on the rides long enough to get my sanity back.

Lowell was on a very special diet at the time. As he couldn't have any sugar, it was a stretch to find anything to feed him at Elitches. We ended up snacking on soft pretzels and a couple of those giant sour pickles. We had already munched on some vegetables and granola on the way down.

After twenty minutes of discussing Victoria Falls, the waterfall in Zimbabwe that had consumed Lowell's attention for several years, we finally got to the front of the line for "The Spider." Lowell was beaming as they strapped us into our little bucket.

I hadn't been to an amusement park since I was a kid. I was a little concerned about whipping my fragile spine around but I didn't want to disappoint Lowell. It wasn't long after we got going that I knew I was in trouble. My stomach did not want to go along for the ride. Convinced that I couldn't go the distance, I started yelling at the other passengers, "Pass it down: I'm sick. Stop the ride."

They stopped the ride all right, with me at the top. I was green by this time. I told Lowell that I was not well and he sat there in deep silence. He was always very concerned and considerate about my welfare. It took them an eternity to unload each car. I didn't make it.

Lowell continued to sit silently as I puked all over myself. There wasn't a square inch of me that was not covered in green slime. Emptying my stomach hadn't brought me any relief either. I still wanted to die.

There were only two or three hundred people waiting in line watching as they finally unloaded us. They stood me up in front of the crowd and hosed me down like an animal. I finally walked away, having lost my lunch and all my dignity on "The Spider." Lowell spoke for the first time since I had announced I was sick. He spun and looked straight at me with the biggest grin I had ever seen him muster and blared, "Wasn't that fun!"

Lowell loved the water and he loved slides, but he was afraid of water slides. I made it my mission one day to help him conquer that fear. God help me! There was a nice water slide at the Loveland Civic Center that was just the right size. It was not too big to be imposing but big enough to grab his interest. I decided to take him there.

We were the only people at the pool that morning, which was a good thing since we spent nearly an hour at the top of the slide discussing his fear and what he thought might happen if he went down the slide. I was so frustrated that I began to cry. Lowell came up behind me and put his hand on my shoulder and stated, "Don't cry, Denise. I'll go down." I was deeply touched. This child had the heart of Jesus. But as much as he wanted to ease my pain, he couldn't overcome his fear.

I asked the lifeguard to turn the water in the slide off. Lowell and I went down the slide several times. He thought that was great fun, but when the lifeguard turned the water back on, Lowell's fear came right back. I finally asked the lifeguard to turn the water off, and when we got halfway down the slide to turn the water back on. He could see that Lowell loved and trusted me and agreed.

Lowell was sitting in my lap as we started down the slide. He heard the water rushing behind me and looked at me with great horror, as if to say, "What have you done?" I began to have doubts after seeing his face. Maybe this would traumatize him too much.

He hit the water and scrambled for the side of the pool. He couldn't get out fast enough. I tried to get to him so I could talk to him about his fear, but I couldn't catch him. He was already on his way back up the slide. For the next two hours he couldn't climb the steps to the top fast enough. I had started a loop that would take over our lives for the next five years.

For example, besides dealing with the reference to water slides every thirty seconds in our conversations, I found myself climbing a fence in Las Vegas in the middle of the winter to get a picture of a water slide that was closed for the season to send to Lowell. Another winter, he and I climbed a fence in three feet of snow to look at a water slide in Sparks, Nevada. I had created a monster.

One day we headed to Colorado Springs for a weekend outing, about a three-hour drive. The weather was very bad and we hit a blizzard about halfway there. We were traveling on Interstate 25, a major freeway, and I couldn't even see the front of the car because the fog and the snow were so thick.

I was trying to find a safe place to pull off when the car started spinning. We did a full three-sixty in traffic, yet managed not to hit anyone or anything. When the car finally came to a stop, I sat in horrified silence trying to get my heart to start up again. I had almost forgotten that Lowell was there when he piped up, "So, you want to go to Water World?" I wanted to smack him, but as usual I just laughed. The stress drained out of me.

Lowell was a savant in several areas. He could remember dates and was incredible with geography. After I moved to Nevada, I sent him a map of Reno before he flew out to visit me. By the time he landed he knew the city better than I. He told me how to get to my house, having never been there before.

One year, with his family's blessings, Lowell and I had arranged to spend Christmas in a cabin in the mountains that belonged to Kurt, one of my students. Kurt drove us up there a few days before our trip so that we could see where it was and drop off our food.

For our vacation we were planning to park the car at the base of the mountain and cross-country ski to the cabin with our packs on our backs. My pack was full of Christmas presents for Lowell that the students had donated.

At the time, Lowell was having some problems at school because of his swearing in class. He got a lot of attention when he blurted out obscenities. I would let an inappropriate word fly now and then myself. I think using obscenities is one way to express pent-up rage. Lowell and I each had our share.

We made a pact. We could say whatever we wanted while we were alone together in the mountains. We agreed that it was okay to "get it out" as long as we weren't offending anyone. Once we got back to the car, if one of us said something "bad" the other was to punch the offender on the arm. I parked the car at the base of the mountains and we strapped on our skis.

My students had thrown me a wonderful Christmas party the night before. It was to be my last Christmas with them and with Lowell, for I was closing my school and leaving the state. This particular morning I was very tired, a bit hung over, and quite emotional.

Lowell was a great skier, much better than I. The only problem was that he didn't register pain. He could fly down a hill and smack into a tree and not recognize that he was injured, so I was always a little on edge when we skied.

We had been skiing for several hours. Sundown was approaching, I was exhausted, and I was sure we were lost. I had kept my mouth shut thus far because I didn't want to alarm Lowell. I finally admitted, "Lowell, we're lost. I don't know where the cabin is and I don't want us out here after sundown. We'll have to go back to the car, put the chains on and try to drive to the cabin."

"Gee, Denise," he innocently replied, "I know exactly where it is." He took off skiing and had us at the cabin in twenty minutes. From then on, Lowell was the navigator for all our excursions.

The next day was Christmas Eve. We rose early and I fixed us a nice hot bowl of oatmeal. Lowell was great to cook for; he would eat anything without complaining. For that matter, this skinny kid was a virtual eating machine. I often wondered if he had a tapeworm.

Lowell looked up from his oatmeal with a big grin on his face and declared, "This is some good shit!" It had begun. We swore like sailors for three days and had a ball.

We chopped down a Christmas tree for the cabin that day and decorated it with pine cones, a few Christmas bulbs we found, and some decorations that we made out of aluminum foil. All the while we talked about Santa Claus. Lowell was concerned that Santa would never find us so deep in the mountains. I assured him that I had let the Clauses know where we'd be spending Christmas.

It was a full moon that night. We skied down this beautiful, white, tree-lined path, singing Christmas carols as we skied. There was no denying the existence of God that night; the scene was breathtaking! I was overcome with emotion.

Lowell was a ways ahead of me as per usual. I could feel that he was enjoying the moment as much as I was. He looked over his shoulder and shouted, "Hey, Denise."

"What?" I hollered back.

"Fuck you!" he shouted as he laughed. I about fell off my skis. What a moment!

After Lowell fell asleep that night, I quietly plucked the gifts from my pack and placed them under the tree. I couldn't wait to see him discover them.

He was up for quite a while the next morning before he noticed the gifts. I thought I would explode with anticipation. They finally caught his eye, and he dove at the tree. He was tearing them open with great delight when he suddenly stopped dead. He became morose.

He looked sadly at me and whimpered, "But there aren't any for you." I explained to him that I had asked Santa to leave mine in Loveland because I didn't want to haul them all down the mountain. He thought that over for a moment and then went gleefully back to his gifts. I went outside and cried. This child continued to burrow his way into the depths of my soul. Thank you, Lowell!

When this magical vacation was over, we headed back to town. Lowell tested me a few times on the way to see if the no cursing rule was going to be enforced, receiving a few friendly pounds on the arm. His teachers told me that he managed to hold his tongue after that. They were quite overwhelmed by my methods, but nothing they had tried had worked.

My leaving Colorado was very traumatic for Lowell. He started a terrible downward spiral. I still carry a lot of guilt about that. I was the only person in Lowell's life, other than family, who spent time with him out of choice. Everyone else was paid. Our bond was very deep and he suffered greatly after I left. So did I.

Sometimes he would call five times a week, sometimes five times a day. Anyone who ever lived with me after I left Colorado, be it lover or roommate, had a relationship with Lowell. He wanted to talk to me, but if I wasn't home he would engage whoever was unlucky enough to have answered the phone until they found a way to break loose.

The first time he came to visit me in Reno, the airline lost his luggage, luggage that held his all-important medications. He was sixteen at the time, I think, and he had been on meds for thirteen years. He had terrible facial ticks as a result of the constant stream of medications.

I was told that the medications were to regulate his behaviors, and that he could become harder and harder to handle and possibly violent without these drugs.

When his suitcase didn't arrive I began to panic, remembering the now infamous Comet incident. One morning Lowell had been home alone when the rage that was sedated inside him found its way to the surface. He took a can of Comet and flung it, amongst other things, all over his parent's kitchen. It took days to clean it up.

The airline was quite nonchalant about the whole thing. Lowell's bag was apparently vacationing in Phoenix. They would let us know if and when it arrived.

I parked Lowell in the waiting area and went in to speak to the lost-luggage gal. "I'll tell you what, lady. You get that luggage here now or I am going to leave him here with you!" Lowell was already notorious; the flight attendant who had spent the last four hours with him was having a nervous breakdown in the back room. They would get on it ASAP, I was told.

Fortunately I didn't live far from the airport. We decided to go home and wait for their call. It was a long afternoon. Lowell popped off the couch every few minutes and said, "Okay, let's go get my bag." I had to keep explaining that it hadn't arrived yet. By bedtime we still had no luggage.

Lowell's mother was trying to arrange to have his prescription called into a pharmacy in Reno, but it was a weekend and she couldn't get his doctor on the phone. So far Lowell was doing fine. I, on the other hand, was a nervous wreck. His luggage finally showed up late the next afternoon. By this time Lowell was not only doing fine, he was doing great. He was calmer and quieter, and his facial ticks were not nearly as pronounced as usual.

I called his mother, Deb. We discussed it and decided to let Lowell keep going without the medications. It was the first time in thirteen years that his liver had gotten a break from the continual flow of dangerous chemicals. It was also the first time that he had experienced any relief from the constant involuntary twitching and convulsing of his facial muscles. It changed him significantly. Thank God for small disasters. More on Lowell later...

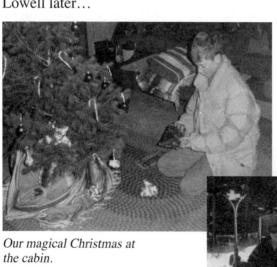

Our magical Christmas at the cabin.

Lowell getting ready to ski the mountain at Virginiadale.

FOOD FOR THOUGHT...

I learned so much from Lowell that I couldn't begin to recite it all here. I guess the most significant thing that Lowell gave me was unconditional love. He could not have cared less about my physical beauty or my bank account. He loved me, just the way I was.

That love is, in my opinion, the most transforming gift there is. It is a shame that we label people like Lowell "disabled." Could it be that those of us who can't experience love and wonder like Lowell can are the disabled ones?

JUST FOR FUN...

Rainman, Forest Gump and Monica Lewinski decided to go shopping, but couldn't decide on a destination. Rainman says, "Hey, let's go to K-Mart and buy some underwear."

Forest Gump whimpers, "No, I want to go to Russell Stover's and buy a box of chocolates."

Monica pipes up with "I've got it. We can cruise over to Frederick's of Hollywood and pick up some chocolate underwear!"

An original (Sorry, Monica. Bless your heart, you got crucified for reflecting our behaviors back at us!)

THE BODYGUARD

After ten years of living in a Do-Jang, parked in the same place, this rolling stone was ready for something new. Tae Kwon-Do had been good to me. But I was thirsty for some fresh knowledge and experiences, and my students deserved better. I was losing my zest for teaching the same things over and over. It showed in my work.

I was at a friend's house watching television one afternoon when I saw an advertisement for a bodyguard school. It looked like something out of a James Bond movie — cars spinning, guns aimed, agents sneaking around.

I had done some unofficial bodyguard work accompanying my professional gambler friends back and forth to Las Vegas (that's another book). These guys traveled with $30,000 in cash on them or more. I learned a lot assisting them in staying out of harm's way.

I already had plenty of knowledge, skills and experience to get a bodyguard job, but the school looked like one hell of an adventure. I called the number advertised on the screen.

The course entailed six months of classes at Denver Business College, a two-week residency program in Aspen at the headquarters of Executive Security International, and $10,000. I couldn't imagine how I would pay for the program but I took the entrance exam anyway.

The business college rep informed me that I had out-scored 98 percent of the applicants who had ever applied to Denver Business College, so I could look forward to some grants and loans. I started school in May of 1989. I was planning to close my Tae Kwon-Do school and pursue my new career by Christmas, sooner if an opportunity came along.

I loved my class. There was only one other woman out of thirty students in it, and she was an associate of mine, Eva Graziano. Eva had also out-scored the pack at Denver Business College.

The remainder of the class consisted of ex-military guys, security guards, a cop, a former pro football player, a Green Beret, some miscellaneous folks and a CIA guy who brought a lot of intrigue to our group. The instructor, Jim Johanson, was an ex-cop who really made this classroom rock. We studied: Executive Security, Escape and Evasion Driving, Defensive Shooting, Observational Psychology, Antiterrorism, Presidential Security, and more.

Practicing Presidential Security techniques was especially interesting to me. The mass effort that it takes to protect the most at-risk person on the planet is like a ballet, an intricately planned dance around one continuously moving target.

Presidential security requires a monster effort towards prevention — gathering information about the location and the people that the principal is going to be exposed to ahead of time. We were taught at ESI "If you have to draw your gun — you've failed. Prevention is everything!" They called it front work.

To practice these skills, we were divided into groups and given an assignment to gather information about the car dealership next to the school. Jim wanted us to find out the dimensions of the lot, the hours of operation, the workings of their security system, who watches the place, etc. We huddled in teams around the room, excitedly discussing our strategies. This was a competition to see who could get the best information. The guys in my group were all focused on espionage. I had a different plan. We split up and agreed to meet at a designated place and time to compile our data.

I always went to class dressed up. I was the only single woman in a closed space with thirty men for six months. "There's got to be one decent guy in here," I thought. But this day I was going to focus on the men at the dealership. It just so happened I had on my best dress.

My plan was to sweet-talk somebody over there into giving me the information I needed. I decided to just head over and wing it; I would come up with the right story when I met them. I made a Hollywood entrance as I waltzed through the front door. The head "dude" came bounding up to me, grabbed my hand, kissed it and welcomed me to his dealership. "This is going to be like taking candy from a baby," I giggled to myself. The story came to me. I'd tell him the truth!

"Hi!" I chirped, flashing my friendliest smile. "I'm Denise. I'm in the ESI program across the street." ESI was famous for these little games. The local businesses were usually notified so they didn't shoot any of the students. "We're supposed to gather information about your business. There are twenty-eight guys crawling around outside as we speak. Wanna help me out?"

He was a happily married puppy dog who just liked to flirt. He told me everything down to their bank account and had a good laugh as he walked me back to the door. When our group presented our findings, there were some complaints from our competitors that we (meaning I) had cheated. I pointed out to them and Jim, the judge, that I had merely used what tools and imagination I had available to me to produce the desired results.

Wasn't that what a good soldier or front person is supposed to do? Jim agreed.

On Fridays we had show and tell. We had the whole school to ourselves because the other classes let out early on that day. Everybody liked to bring a favorite weapon. The CIA guy brought all kinds of interesting stuff: grenades, bazookas, AK47s, spears and such.

He was a strange man and had seen a lot of horror. He told a story of being in combat in the Middle East. He had grabbed a guy by the hair and was planning to slit his throat but accidentally beheaded him instead. He got this crazed look on his face as he talked about holding the head in his hand, just inches from his face. It was quite apparent that he had not healed from all the traumas he had experienced. Yet he seemed to thrive on it. It made his juices flow.

One day he disappeared off the face of the planet. Neither his family, nor his roommate, nor the school knew what had happened to him. We all suspected that he had been called out by the CIA and concocted numerous tales of what he might be up to.

I had started seeing one of the guys in my class. Ron was younger than I and recovering from breaking up with the love of his life — another Denise. Although he was twenty-three to my thirty-two, in many categories of life he was more grown up than I was. He was tough, determined, patriotic, honest and kind, which was fortunate because he had his hands full with me. Ron walked with me through some really dark times.

We started out our relationship however, going through this school together, which was a gas. The program included a lot of the Bond-like escapades. We spent four days at the racetrack with a professional racecar driver and an ex-cop who taught us how to race cars, spin them, wreck them, evade them, jump out of them, and maneuver them in a motorcade.

We spent two days racing around the track with a glass of water suspended in a drink holder on the door, learning how to perform maneuvers at a designated speed, without spilling the water. We learned to spin cars around a hundred and eighty degrees and to perform three-sixties. We ran maneuvers full speed in reverse. We got to ram other vehicles, and more. Man we had a ball!

Additionally, we put in four days on the shooting range. We were required to pass a target-shooting test before going on to the more advanced maneuvers. I had not done any shooting before enrolling in ESI, so they recommended that I buy the gun that many police forces now use, a Glock. We learned to shoot from a moving vehicle, and how to walk into a shooting gallery with a "principal" to protect. We were shooting live ammunition at moving targets over each other's heads.

There was a day of playing commandos with paint balls in a mock combat scenario. That was a kick, but the darn things really stung when they hit you. I had on several layers of clothing and a thick coat and still had bruises from each hit.

One game I really liked. All the weapons were placed in a pile and we formed two teams. We had to jog in place, then run to the weapons table carrying a tire, grab a weapon, hit a target, put the weapon and the tire back and then tag our teammate. This game helped us learn to use a variety of weapons and experience how heart rate and heavy breathing would affect our aim. It was a brilliant training technique.

One day they had forgotten to bring a water supply for the range. We had been running, shooting and sweating in the sun for hours. I stumbled up to the instructor and mumbled, "I think you better take this loaded gun off my hip, I'm going to pass out." He did and I did. I came around in the ambulance after some intravenous fluids.

We did more espionage and front work assignments in Aspen, where we were in danger of being attacked with paint balls by the staff on the way to class each morning.

ESI brought in an instructor who had many years experience on the streets in emergency medicine. He explained the human body like a car, having a beautiful rap that broke it all down in simple layman's terms. Almost all the guys had some mechanical skills, so it was really meaningful to them.

The shooting, driving, commandos and playing doctor was a hoot, but I was surprised to find that the four days of classroom study we sat through in the residency program was as exhilarating as the hands on training.

The observational psychology class was my personal favorite. A renowned, published authority on the subject taught that unit. I'm sorry I don't remember his name. We were given a test at the beginning of the day and again at the end to see how much we had learned. I scored very high the first time. I had taught observational psychology to every group I had trained in personal safety, but this guy had an amazing tool.

He flashed a picture on a screen for 1/25th of a second. We then had to determine the mood of the subject we had briefly seen — were they happy, sad, angry, fearful, etc. It is astounding how much you can tell about somebody after just getting a glance at them. Secret Service agents are highly skilled at this.

We watched the Reagan assassination attempt over and over along with a couple of other famous attempts on world leaders' lives. What was most disturbing was the realization that these events had generally been preventable.

When President Reagan stepped out into the public that day, the Secret Service agent who was to walk on Mr. Reagan's left was in the bathroom. We watched a tape of what he would have seen had he been in his rightful place in the formation. He would have seen a jubilant crowd of people excitedly waiting to see the President — and one very morose guy standing alone in a giant overcoat with his arms crossed. The agent who went to the bathroom was trained to notice these things. He would be expected to keep an eye on a man like Hinkley — making a strong argument that the shooting could have been prevented.

Jack MacGeorge was my favorite instructor. He was an ex-Secret Service/Demolitions expert who had started his own security business. He had worked with many presidents and political heavyweights and had an endless litany of fascinating stories. I especially liked the one about Harvey's Hotel and Casino in Lake Tahoe.

A gambler had a $250,000 marker out at Harvey's, a "marker" being money he had borrowed from the house to gamble on. The powers-that-be of the casino called in his loan. They wanted their money now! The gambler didn't have it, so he devised a plan.

He built a bomb the size of a mainframe computer, threw a tarp over it, and walked it in the front door of the casino on a dolly, just after office hours. He had on overalls with a company insignia on them and told security he was delivering a computer. They signed for it and let him park it in the office area. He then went home and called the "big boys" demanding that they forgive his debt and throw in another $4.75 million or he was going to blow the place to kingdom come.

Jack MacGeorge's team was called in, as well as everybody who was anybody from every agency imaginable. Apparently the local law enforcement Joes at the time were "Andy and Barney of Mayberry" types. Jack's team examined the bomb in awe. This guy was a genius, and he had created a monster. Their report to the folks at Harvey's said, "Pay the man!"

Andy and Barney and the boys were sure that they could disarm this thing with a technique that requires great accuracy — shooting a stream of water through the bomb like the slice of a knife. Jack's team reviewed the plan (which can be used in some cases) and repeated, "Pay the man!" Andy and Barney blew a hole in the casino you could drive a train through. No one was hurt, and Harvey's got a nice insurance settlement that allowed them to remodel. Perhaps Andy and Barney weren't so dumb?

Jack also taught us how to pick locks and gather sensitive information. We listened to him for sixteen hours a day. I could have sat still for twenty. He was fascinating.

The founder of Executive Security International is also a very fascinating man. Bob Duggan has worked with the Secret Service, the CIA, the Navy Seals and the FBI. He also handled the Pope's visit to Denver.

Bob had been a terrorist at one point and then chose to change his life. He went to the American government and offered, "I can teach you how a terrorist thinks." It helps to crawl into the head of the guy you're trying to protect against.

Bob is a highly accomplished martial arts instructor. He taught a self-defense class and some weapon-disarming techniques that I ended up sharing with laymen and law enforcement alike. The moves were brilliant, based on the laws of physics and people's proven abilities and reaction times under duress.

ESI was truly an adventure. I learned a lot there that applied to many areas in my life and received a ton of validation and esteem from the experience. I highly recommend it. You don't have to want to be in security to sign up. If you can afford it, it is a life-altering opportunity to stretch yourself.

Eva and I tied three other students for second place in the class standing. Bob made a speech about how he had underestimated us gals and how impressed he was with our performance. He gifted us each with a novel about a female bodyguard. We were off to seek work amongst the rich and famous, we hoped.

After closing my school, Ron and I decided that we would market ourselves as a team and go wherever the work was. We received a call from ESI right away. There was a newspaper strike in St. Paul, Minnesota. The paper needed people to guard the principals of the newspaper and do some general strike work. It paid $100 a day apiece, plus room and board, but we had to commit to three months. These strikes generally drag on forever.

We decided that it would be a great opportunity to pay off our school loans and get some capital to start out on. The hitch was that they wanted us in St. Paul in twenty-four hours.

After moving all our belongings into storage, we gave up our apartment, settled all our affairs and jumped on a plane. Many long, tedious days lay ahead, often in the bitter cold, but we were excited about this new adventure and having some money for a change. And don't forget, I love those changes of venue.

We were part of a group of about sixty security people whom the security company had flown in from all over the country. We gathered a few hours after landing for our orientation meeting. We were all buzzing with anticipation. Who would get the executive security positions and who would be the grunts?

"Good evening, gentlemen and ladies. I appreciate the effort you all made to be here on such short notice. The good news is you are all going to get paid tonight. The bad news is that they settled the strike while you were in the air."

They reimbursed us for our airfare and paid us a couple of hundred dollars a piece for our trouble. Ron and I headed back to Denver the next day. Jobless and homeless, we packed the truck and headed west. Time for another adventure.

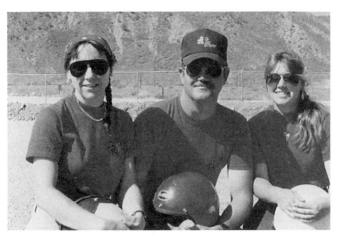

Me, Jim (our instructor) and Eva on the track at ESI.

FOOD FOR THOUGHT...

I really enjoyed this period of my life. For an excitement junky, ESI was awesome. I have shared what I learned there with cops and agencies all over the country who deal in abuse prevention. Good front work assists me in every category of my life. I find that it is easier to walk into any situation with confidence if I have done my homework, proving that age-old Girl Scout motto, "Be prepared."

JUST FOR FUN...

"Good morning, Mr. President. (Bill Clinton was still President when I wrote this book. The editing process can take longer than several presidencies.) My name is Denise, and I'll be your bodyguard from now on sir."

"Where's Bubba, my regular guy?" Mr. Clinton asked.

"He's been reassigned, sir, but I can try to locate him if you like,"

"I want Bubba back. He's the only person I trust with my life," the president declared.

"I understand, sir. It's just that I out-performed him on the range, so I was given his position."

With interest and amazement, the president inquired, "You out-shot Bubba? That's amazing!"

"Well actually, sir, I never hit the target, but I went three days without taking a piss."

"Congratulations, miss, you're hired!"

STUCK IN NEVADA AGAIN

Ron and I headed for Beverly Hills. Since the most important ingredient for finding work as a bodyguard is rich people, it seemed like a wise choice. We found an ex-Beverly Hills cop who wanted to put us to work as soon as we got settled. He had started his own bodyguard business and was plugged in to the stars. The problem was that it took several thousand dollars just to get into an apartment in L.A. and more to get a phone, heat, running water and electricity. We didn't have enough to get a place, so we decided to go to Reno, Nevada. We could easily get a security job at a casino and make enough money to go back to L.A. in a matter of months.

Getting a job in security didn't take an act of God. The standing joke was, if you have a pulse and a social security number, you're hired. Ron and I were more qualified than half the heads of security in Nevada.

I got a job at Circus Circus and Ron was hired at the Eldorado. Together we had spent $20,000 to get an education in the protection field and we were now gainfully employed, schlepping around casinos showing drunks the door for $6 an hour. Yippee.

Circus Circus was particularly excited about my rape prevention background. I was to find out later that they had had a number of rape claims on the property in the five months prior to my coming on board.

Out of one hundred security officers at Circus Circus, only a handful were women. I was treated with a lot of respect, though, because of my training with ESI. I was also deemed quite valuable for my report-writing skills. Casino security is also all about prevention — preventing litigation. If you could write a detailed incident report that would cover the casino's tail in court, you were a valuable commodity. I could and I was, for a while anyway.

Friday night of Memorial Day weekend I was walking the beat in the garage. I had been on the job five months by then. We changed posts every hour so that everybody got to do a little of everything. I liked walking the garage. I got to be alone and outside, moving. It was a welcome relief after many hours sitting and checking I.D.s or guarding a bucket of change.

All of a sudden my walkie-talkie was abuzz with activity. I listened closely to the transmissions going back and forth between one very excited security officer and the dispatcher. Although they were very careful not to say so on the air, I knew immediately that someone had been raped. Breaking company policy, I took off running.

I was the second officer on the scene. The one who had generated all the radio traffic had taken off after the assailant. I entered the hotel room and found a very distraught middle-aged woman. I asked her name. She told me "Sandy." (Not her real name.) I closed the door and began the difficult task of trying to get some information out of her.

One minute she was calm and collected, answering my questions with ease; the next moment she was bouncing off the walls, raging mad and talking suicide. We formed a bond right away.

Although I did not have the authority to do so, I took over the scene. I locked the door and let the dispatcher know that I would be handling this woman. They complained a little at first, but then realized that it was in the best interest of the victim. I was the one most qualified to help her. Little did I know that this woman, and this incident, would consume the next three years of my life.

I had gotten bits and pieces of the story from Sandy and eventually I was able to put most of the puzzle together. She was a local and worked for a rental car agency. It was the first night that she had ever spent apart from her husband in 26 years of marriage. They had been fighting and she decided to spend the night in town. She was able to get a free room from Circus Circus through her company.

Sandy had been playing some slots, sipping wine, just relaxing. She was an attractive woman and was getting more attention than she wanted from some foreign man in the casino, so she decided to head for her room, but she got confused on the casino floor. A young black man approached her and asked if she was lost. He was with an older couple whom he introduced as his aunt and uncle. He was sweet and polite, like the kids that worked under her every day. He offered to show her where the elevators were. Sandy didn't give it a thought.

When they got to the elevator banks, Sandy thanked him for his kindness and stepped onto the elevator. She told him that she could find it from there. As the doors closed he stepped in with her saying that he wanted to make sure she got to her room safely. They had a nice chat in the elevator.

Upon arriving at her floor Sandy thanked him warmly again, but he followed her down the hall. She was too naive to be frightened, but she was getting a little annoyed. When she got to her door she realized that maybe he was expecting a tip. She had a five dollar bill in the bucket of change she had been carrying. She handed it to the young man and thanked him again. He turned and headed down the hall as she fumbled to open her door.

As she was fumbling with the key she heard her phone ringing. She was anxious to get in and answer it as she was hoping it was her husband. She opened the door and lunged at the phone. It turned out to be the man who had been hustling her in the casino. He had gotten her name from her nametag, which she had forgotten to remove after work, and called her room from the lobby. Sandy assured the man that she wasn't interested and hung up the phone. She spun around to find the young black kid standing in her room.

"What are you doing here?" Sandy asked, more incredulous than scared. He came over to her and started to kiss her. She pushed him away, "I'm old enough to be your mother, for God's sake. What are you doing?"

The encounter became violent. The rapist ripped the phone from the wall and threatened to bash her head in with it. Sandy submitted and the attack was over in a matter of minutes. The assailant escaped down the fire stairs and was on the sidewalk running in seconds. He was never found. We later determined, from examining past incident reports, that this same team, meaning the supposed aunt and uncle and nephew, had committed numerous crimes in the hotel towers.

The Reno police were notified. Officer Snyder responded to the scene. He was a real gem. Officer Snyder was the finest police officer I have ever worked with in rape crisis. He was very considerate of Sandy's needs. I felt that Sandy trusted him right away and was relieved. It was about 2 a.m. when he and I escorted Sandy the few blocks to St. Mary's Hospital. She had agreed to go through the rape exam.

At St. Mary's, I stayed in the room with her and Officer Snyder waited outside the door. This man wasn't just on duty. He was deeply touched by the trauma this woman was going through. His job was to get her to fill out a detailed police report on the assault. Circus Circus also wanted a detailed report from me and one from Sandy. I kept telling them all, "In due time. Let's get her through this ordeal at the hospital first."

At one point Sandy went flying out of the examining room screaming and carrying on. I indicated to Officer Snyder that I could handle it, so he let me chase her down. I ended up catching her outside and rocking her in my arms as she talked suicide. She was falling apart, but agreed to give everybody the reports they wanted if they would just leave her alone with me. Officer Snyder thought that would be fine. He gave me the paperwork and explained what he needed. He also gave me a time frame. Could we get this filled out in the next few hours? I assured him I would get it handled.

I talked to my bosses at Circus Circus several times while we were at the hospital. They were trying to reach Sandy's husband but couldn't, so they were going to fix her a fresh room to stay in until we could find someone to take her home. She was not to be left alone. I radioed them that Officer Snyder had turned her over to me and that I would be walking her back to Circus Circus in a few moments. They said they would have someone meet us at the door with a key to the new room.

My supervisor and a lady I didn't know met us at the door. My supervisor gave me the key and the new room number. The lady was the claims agent for Circus Circus. She was shoving a microphone and tape recorder in Sandy's face before we even got through the door.

Sandy was pretty much catatonic at this point. She had her head down, staring at the ground. She had nothing to say. I sure as hell did, though! I told this woman that her actions were totally out of line and not at all in keeping with the way the police asked me to handle this case. I told her that she had no idea what had gone on at the hospital and that Sandy just wanted to be alone with me. I assured her that Sandy would give all the statements they wanted once she felt up to it. Much to my amazement, the woman and my supervisor turned and walked away.

I took Sandy up to the new room and we settled in. A few minutes later there was a knock at the door. It was about 4 a.m. by then. I opened the door to find my supervisor there with a strange look on his face. He had become a personal friend of mine. So when the Head of Security stepped up to the door I was pretty sure what was about to happen next. Security guards, all male, kept coming out of the woodwork.

Sandy was told that I was being fired and that I would have to leave. They asked her if she wanted them to find another woman to come stay with her. She started to cry and said that she wanted me to stay with her. The Head of Security, Ray Lopez, sat down on the bed next to Sandy and put his hand on her thigh, hardly a welcome gesture to a woman who has just been brutally raped. He reiterated that I had to leave but that they would find someone else to comfort her. I was stripped of my badge, radio and I.D. and escorted off the property.

Up until that point Sandy had never considered suing anyone. As she was to tell it, the actual rape had just been a few ugly minutes out of her life; she could have recovered from that. But what Circus Circus did to her was the real rape, and she would never recover from that!

Sandy and I filed a joint lawsuit against Circus Circus. She was suing for negligence and I was suing for wrongful termination. Eventually our cases were severed. My case was put on hold until some state Supreme Court case was settled. Sandy's case became bigger than life.

Unbeknownst to Sandy, the door of her room had been broken. It was supposed to close and lock automatically behind her. It hadn't, allowing the assailant to just waltz into her room. The Circus Circus security regulations specified that each hotel tower was to be toured by security every hour, twenty-four hours a day. The tower her room was in had not been toured by security at all that day. The assailant had been stopped twice in the casino and asked for I.D. He didn't have any. According to the casino's own security policies, the young man should have been walked to the property line and warned not to return. I was the only one who had gotten that treatment that night. Sandy had plenty of grounds for her case.

That story is another whole book in itself. For the next three years Sandy endured an endless, vicious attack from the system that she had looked to for justice. She went to court time and again and lost every battle.

I joined the Sexual Assault Advocacy Team in Reno to help other victims, and I ran to Sandy whenever she called. I spent many sleepless nights racing to her home in the foothills when she would call me talking suicide. Her life was a nightmare and I felt obligated to stand behind her, even though I was powerless to help her fight the system that was beating her down. The fact that I had manifested Sandy and more rape crisis work into my life at that time would prove to be quite profound.

Ron and I had moved into town by now. The first job I landed after Circus Circus was with Brinks Armored Car as an armed messenger. The driver got $6 an hour and I received $6.25 because I was the one who would have to get out of the armored car and possibly get shot at.

The company policy was: if I ran into trouble while outside the truck, the driver was to leave me there and take off. Apparently, the contents of the truck were deemed more valuable than my life. My first day on the job, I picked up a clear plastic bag from the Peppermill Casino that contained one million dollars in cash. By the end of the day I had five million in the back of the truck with me. Twice a week we would head out to the desert and pick up $250,000 worth of gold from the mines. It was an interesting job, but Brinks was struggling to compete in Reno and soon went out of business there.

I bounced from job to job after that, working security and then cocktailing in the casinos. I was much happier being in a service position where I could generate tips, but I was generally treated like crap everywhere I worked. That's how the casinos keep from paying high wages to senior employees. They try their damnedest to run you off.

In the midst of all this chaos in my life I got a call from my cousin Ruthie. She had never called me just to chat, so I knew something was up. Ruthie stammered and stumbled over her tongue until she finally just said it:

"Your father died last night."

The first thing that came to mind was "Ding dong the witch is dead!" It had been over twelve years since I had disowned my parents. I had often wondered how I would feel if one of them died and we hadn't healed our problems. Now I would find out. I had a lot of thoughts that day, but I can't say that I had any real feelings. I was numb.

I set out to find my sister to give her the news. It was Christmas time and she usually spent Christmas deep in the mountains of New York with her husband and a family that she had been close to since college. It took an hour's worth of work with the help of directory assistance to finally locate her.

Paula seemed much more shocked and overwhelmed than I was as she excitedly announced the news to the gathering in the background. I wondered why I didn't feel more. It reminded me of the day Uncle Woody, my father's only sibling, had died. I was seven.

Everybody was hysterical and crying. I adored this man, yet hard as I tried to come up with an emotion, I couldn't even shed a tear.

This day I couldn't even decide on an emotion, let alone express one, but I did sense a feeling of peace coming to me. Perhaps my father's death would bring some closure to the past. Instead it was to open "Pandora's Box." I got what I prayed for. I was going to learn how to feel.

The first very profound feeling that came to me was that I missed my brother. I had never wanted to lose Sam, but he had opted to join forces with my parents when I had disowned them. At that time he had written me a scathing letter saying, "How could you do this to our family?"

My thoughts were "What family?"

Our family life had seemed like "Every man to himself," or "Whose side are you on today?" The concept that we had ever been a family was foreign to me.

I had heard that my mother and my brother had become very close over the years, so I knew exactly where he would be. I called my mother's house. I had gotten her number from my cousin.

Sam answered the phone. On one hand he seemed happy to hear from me, on the other hand he was angry. He didn't want my mother traumatized any more than she was. He said, "What were you going to do if Mom answered the phone?"

I tentatively replied, "Talk to her, I suppose."

Sam told me about my father's death. He had turned seventy-three that week, I believe, seeming quite healthy and still golfing daily. David had gone out to get the paper. When he bent down to pick it up, he was in trouble. My mother convinced him to go to the hospital. The doctor told him that he had experienced a mild heart attack, and that he would either be just fine or he would have a massive heart attack within the next twenty-four hours. Sam says that David lay there in utter terror until he had a massive heart attack the next day and died. I have never thought about it before this moment, but it strikes me as I am writing this, how profound it is that my father basically died of fear. Good job, Doc. I suspect you scared him to death!

Sam also told me that David had a lot to say about me on his deathbed. Apparently he was quite bitter that I wasn't there and that I had never come back to the family. I wonder what I would have done had they called me the night before? I don't know.

My brother called back before long and said that my mother wanted to buy me a car. I could fly down to Texas, pick out something and drive it back. It seemed like a great opportunity to heal some old wounds. I sincerely appreciated her gesture and I needed a vehicle. I flew down first. Ron joined me a week later.

Seeing my brother's face at the Houston airport was wonderful. He has a sweet, loving essence about him. When I saw him I was immediately reminded of something he had once done that had touched me deeply.

Sam loved the ladies and was usually on the prowl. One day he was laying his best lines on a hostess in a restaurant when she started sobbing violently. She told him that she had recently been raped and she could not handle his advances.

Sam worked his tail off and earned the money to buy her a beautiful diamond necklace. He went back to the restaurant, saying as he presented the lovely gift to her, "I just want you to know that all men aren't like that." He left and never bothered her again.

It was like old times. I spent several days with him and his fiancée in Houston. They were very generous with me and treated me like royalty. Then came the day they drove me the three hours or so to my mother's house outside of Austin. I was so nervous about seeing my mother that I thought I would faint. She opened the door and threw her arms around me. She was thrilled with how great I looked. Of course, I still felt that I looked like a cow, but in reality I had a very nice figure.

We had a pleasant visit, although I was very nervous the whole time. I had never seen this house, just the empty lot before they had built on it, yet I recognized half the belongings in it. My parents had not wasted much money over the years on new furniture or knick-knacks. It was strange to be around all this old stuff.

Ron and I picked out a nice minivan and headed off on a trip. We had started a company selling custom made, color-changing T-shirts. Now that we had some good wheels we could go on the road. Unfortunately, the van only lasted six months before dropping the engine in nowhere California. We had maintained an apartment in Reno, and as we had spent all of our expense money on the van, we headed home.

I began to feel that something was missing in my life, some piece of myself that I couldn't reach. I started searching. Everywhere I looked I came up with information about sexual abuse. One day, I picked up a book called The Courage to Heal. It had a checklist of more than thirty characteristics or behaviors consistent with survivors of sexual abuse. I answered yes to all but one of the questions. That really confused me, but the more I read the book, the more I felt like the puzzle was coming together. If this had actually happened to me, it would explain a lot of things in my life that had not made sense. It would also give me a place to look to start healing these old wounds. My problem was that repressed memories, if I had any, are not that easy to retrieve. Sometimes they come back spontaneously and sometimes they are gone forever.

Right before I left Loveland I had met a woman whose story had touched me profoundly. Now I knew why she had come into my life. Let's call her Jane.

Jane was in her early forties — beautiful, vibrant and quite friendly. I was killing some time in a restaurant one afternoon and so was she. We struck up a conversation. We were total strangers. I told her about the rape prevention program I was teaching and that the current group of women I was working with were all rape and incest survivors. It was pretty heavy stuff. She shared her story with me.

She thought that she had lived a fairy-tale life until recent months. Her son had become very ill, and he was now on dialysis daily. The strain of her constant worry seemed to have spontaneously brought back some repressed memories. Now that she "owned" these memories again she didn't know how to put her life back together.

Apparently the fairy tale she thought she had lived was a lie. She now had vivid, undeniable memories of her father, a Bible-thumping Baptist preacher, chasing her around the house with knives, and tying her up and raping her. She had been just a child. She told me all this matter-of-factly, as if we were discussing the weather. I was dumbstruck. How could anyone forget something like that, and how could they be so unaffected by it? Another lesson in denial. I invited her to jump into my class. She showed up one day but fled out the door in a matter of minutes. She said that she was "absolutely terrified of facing those old demons." I was overwhelmed with her leaving but didn't really know why.

In that same class there was a woman with multiple personalities who had been the victim of severe, prolonged incest. I learned a lot from her. She was one brave cookie! There was a woman who had been raped by her boss, a woman who had been tackled and molested while out jogging, and the list went on.

I had worked with survivors of sexual abuse for ten years and never even suspected that it might have happened to me. Now I couldn't deny the evidence that it probably had, yet I still had no memories. I tried hypnosis and still didn't find anything. I finally decided to attend a support group for incest survivors, thinking that maybe their stories would trigger something. I felt completely at home there, like I belonged to a sisterhood that truly accepted me for who I was – flaws and all. I was jealous that most of them were so sure what had happened to them. I felt I could deal with the truth if I could just get to it.

Be careful what you pray for, you might just get it! My memories started to come back. I would get a "body memory" first and then a while later get a picture to go with it. Body memories are a fairly well documented phenomenon. The body stores emotional data in its cells as well as physical or pictorial data.

One day I woke up in great terror. My heart was trying to jump out of my chest, I had pain running down my left arm and I was very short of breath. Given my vast family history of heart disease, I was worried. I tried to relax and ride it out, but I was too scared. Finally, I insisted that Ron take me to the hospital.

The ER doctor also thought that I was having a heart attack. He called in a heart specialist and ran $2000 worth of tests in two hours. They knew that I had no insurance and no income so they must have been genuinely concerned. Usually when you tell them you have no insurance, you are out the door with a clean bill of health in five minutes. They found nothing. I was perfectly fine.

That night I experienced my first significant memory. It was not a vivid, video replay that I could embrace fully. It was just a still picture of being sexually assaulted by my father, and the feelings that went with it. I was overcome with fear and grief, but I was also angry. I wanted proof positive. There was plenty of room for doubt here.

A few months later, Ron and I were to relive this whole scenario, but this time it got messy. I was home alone one day when I started bleeding very heavily vaginally. My menstrual periods are usually two days of light bleeding, hardly noticeable. This day I was bleeding like a stuck pig. I finally got undressed and just stood in the bathtub with the cordless phone as I talked to the ER.

When I told them that the bathtub was covered in blood they were prepared to send an ambulance. I told them I would get a friend to bring me right over. My friend Nancy came immediately. I was bleeding so heavily that we were concerned about getting me the two miles to the hospital without destroying her car.

When I arrived at the ER at St. Mary's they gave me a sanitary pad to put on. I laughed and said, "I don't think so." They brought me a hand towel, then a bath towel. Eventually they shoved a blanket between my legs. The ER was covered in blood and these combat-worn doctors and nurses were totally overwhelmed.

The gynecological (GYN) specialist finally arrived. He examined me thoroughly and ran some tests. It was his opinion that I was "healthy as a bear." Except for this fluid loss problem I was having, he couldn't find a thing wrong with me. I was given a drug to stop the bleeding and sent home with strict instructions to come right back if the bleeding started up again.

That night Ron had to go back to work, and I was home alone. I had the most vicious pain shoot up my vagina that I have ever experienced. It frightened me to the bone. I was terrified of having another one. I lay down on the bed and tried to relax. Another freeze frame came to me. In this picture, I was laid out on a table in my room and my father was doing something between my legs. It seemed like he had a vacuum. My suspicion was that he was giving me an abortion. All of a sudden a calm washed over me, draining the fear out of my body.

The next day, however, the bleeding started up again. I went back to the hospital. I told them about the memory or vision or whatever that I had experienced the night before. They were dumbfounded and still had no explanation as to what was happening to me. After telling them my story I was told to relax, as much as one can with a blanket stuck between their legs, and wait for the GYN specialist again. By the time he arrived, I had completely stopped bleeding. He still found nothing wrong with me.

A month later, my sister found an article about these home abortion kits that had been sold underground in the late sixties, early seventies. They attached to a regular home vacuum. My mystery seemed to be unfolding.

After several more months of similar incidents I finally came to believe that I indeed had been sexually violated as a child. I flew to Texas to confront my mother about what I now believed had happened to me. My brother flopped around like a fish out of water, denying that our childhood had been anything but wonderful. His denial was validation for me. Denial is always a red flag that there is some real painful stuff underneath worth lying about or repressing.

At first my mother refused to believe that any such thing had happened. Then she tempered her refusal and said, "If anything like that did happen, I was not aware of it." That was not the whole truth either. In my memories she had been deeply involved. But I was not ready to discuss that with her. That was the day that she told me that I had been an unplanned child. Although she clearly felt terrible as she spoke about it, it wasn't a big deal to me. It was, however, another piece of the puzzle and made me feel a little more whole.

My mother and I agreed to put this topic to rest and move on with our mission of creating a relationship after all these years apart. What she really wanted, though, was for me to adopt the fantasy that I had grown up with Ward and June Cleaver, move on with my life and not talk about any of this ever again. I couldn't do that.

The most damaging thing about sexual abuse is the secret. Many survivors I have met were threatened with their lives: "If you tell anyone, I will kill you!" The secret becomes the monster instead of the abuse. It has been that way for me.

I have long since forgiven my parents and come to peace with what happened and why, but this is the first time I have ever committed to getting my power back from "The Secret." It is the most difficult work I have ever done.

FOOD FOR THOUGHT...

I don't want to believe that my parents were capable of such atrocities, but I can't deny the pictures, feelings and knowing that I have. With each memory that came back, and by walking through each terrifying experience that came with it, I got a piece of myself back. I was beginning to feel more whole.

I want to make it very clear that neither my therapist, nor my hypnotherapist, planted these ideas in my head. I asked Ted Burgess, the hypnotherapist I sought out, if I had been sexually abused. Ted said, "I can't tell you that."

I told him that I wanted to search for my memories. Ted explained, "It doesn't work that way. If indeed you were sexually abused, your memories will surface when you are ready. You can't make it happen." I was never led into these beliefs.

According to the FBI, one in three females and one in five males will be sexually abused in their lifetime. This was not an exclusive club I had joined.

JUST FOR FUN...

Whoa! That was heavy, let's lighten up. Since we're stuck in Nevada, how about a gambling tale? One of the favorite pastimes of gamblers is swapping bad beat stories. A "bad beat" is a poker term describing a situation where you not only lost the pot, but you lost with really good cards. I have a rather unique bad beat story...I won.

It was the first time I had ever played poker for real money. Yung had staked me in a seven-card-stud game at a Denver poker club. Before long I was down to two dollars.

I caught some high, suited cards and decided to go "all-in." That meant that every player on the table who wanted to stay in the hand had to match my two dollars. They could continue to bet after that, but a separate pot would be created.

I ended up with a royal flush, the highest hand you can get in poker. The other players were gambling like crazy, calling and raising every round. I wondered why they were still betting when I obviously had the best hand. I was so naïve about poker that I didn't realize that I couldn't win all the money on the table.

When it was all said and done, they pushed me twelve dollars for my unbeatable royal flush. Some professional poker players have camped at poker tables daily for twenty years and never pulled a royal.

I could whine that I caught a hand that only comes around every twenty-six thousand deals, and I only had two dollars left to gamble on it. Or, I could say that it was a blessing that I turned my last two dollars into twelve so that I could stay in the game. Life is a matter of perspective.

SAVVY!

Ron was a real trooper for standing by me through those dark times. Unfortunately, the relationship didn't make it. I was learning to look at the past with more clarity, and I was becoming able to express my feelings. The army had taught Ron to muscle through his pain, and to deny his emotions — that stuff was for girls. When I couldn't get him to move out of those beliefs, I destroyed the relationship by cheating on him. Ron has since remained a wonderful, supportive friend. I wish him all the best.

Once again, I couldn't escape my karma. The relationship I got into nearly destroyed me. The guy I got involved with emotionally battered me until there was precious little left of Denise. I ended up drinking, smoking cigarettes, doing hard drugs, and gambling, none of which eased my pain. (How's that for sedation!) Thanks to the "crank" (a very toxic form of speed that one snorts) I was doing with my new boyfriend, I managed to take off that last fifteen pounds. The sick thing was that it really did make me happy to be thin, in spite of the fact that I had destroyed my life and my health to do it. I hardly ate, and what I did eat I still purged.

I set out to get my life together, yet again. I had no trouble giving up the crank now that I was thin. It is horrible stuff, akin to snorting Drano. I ditched the boyfriend when he refused to admit that he had a drug problem, and I lost my job as a taxi cab driver (some great stories there for another book).

The cigarettes stayed with me, however, but I hated every single one I smoked. As a person who had dedicated twelve years of my life to martial arts I felt like a failure, but I was afraid of getting fat again if I quit smoking — a reasonable fear, as most people eat more when they quit.

I borrowed $8000 from my mother and decided to quit working in toxic jobs and try to build my rape prevention classes into a full-time business. My mother was very supportive over the next few years. Besides lending me money she also wrote me loving, encouraging letters.

After I suffered numerous failed attempts to market my classes on my own, Jan Clemons came into my life. Jan was the head of the Woman's Center for St. Mary's Hospital in Reno. She recognized the value of my work and set out to establish my program through the hospital. This is the same hospital that had treated my hemorrhaging, and conducted the rape exam on Sandy.

St. Mary's did all the advertising, supplied the room, the mats, some of the props, and fielded the phone calls. All I had to do was show up, collect the money and teach. What I was to find out, however, was that there wasn't enough money or beautiful brochures to overcome the denial. We had a couple of great classes, but all in all we canceled more than I taught due to lack of participants.

I loved teaching this class. Those who showed up got a life-altering experience. They learned how to handle themselves emotionally, verbally, and physically so as not to exude the "victim" energy. They practiced engaging in combat while hauling babies, purses, and groceries, wearing skirts and high-heeled shoes. They were also taught how to fight on the ground in the event they got tackled. And, most important, they learned how to prevent being a target.

But recruiting students was an exhausting task. The denial was so pervasive that for every class I marketed I heard hundreds of comments like "Oh I don't need to do that. Things like that don't happen in my neighborhood." "I can't afford it" was a popular one too, usually from women sporting designer clothes, porcelain nails and a $100 perm. Again, the statistics are that one in three females and one in five males will be sexually abused in their lifetime.

After about six months of this I decided that another change of venue was in order. I couldn't stand Nevada in the first place, and now it was just a huge monument to all my addictions and to denial. People were too busy working, drinking, gambling, smoking and snorting to care about much else.

With $150 in my pocket I loaded my old Saab with all my office supplies and training equipment and headed to the Northwest. I told everybody that I was moving to Seattle. I needed a big city with a crime problem to support my business.

I rolled into Portland, Oregon, at sunrise. It was the most beautiful city I had ever seen. But I had heard that Seattle was even nicer. In my imaginings, Seattle was looking like the "Emerald City" of The Wizard of Oz.

I hit Seattle a few hours later. Maybe I wasn't in the right part of town but it looked like a big ugly city to me. It had been a rough trip and my arm was in excruciating pain. I had spent the week before leaving Nevada digging stumps to make some money. As per usual, I had really overdone it. I found a YMCA in Seattle that lent me some medical supplies and I headed back to Portland. What the hell, I didn't know anybody in either city. I might as well pick the one that I liked.

I was ten miles outside of Portland when the car broke down on the on-ramp to a major freeway. Nobody stopped to help me, but I managed to get the car off the road. I was parked about twenty feet from some railroad tracks and smoke was pouring out of the hood of the car.

I had known that I had electrical problems before I left Nevada but they were intermittent. You know the kind — they start up as soon as you get a block away from the mechanic who just told you that the car is fine and charged you $200 for that verdict.

I had about $120 to my name, hadn't slept in two days, hadn't eaten much, was in pain, and didn't know a soul within 700 miles. I couldn't imagine how I was going to get through this and I was too tired and discouraged to have any emotional reserves left.

Hearing a train in the distance, I began to consider suicide. Hurling myself in front of the train would probably be a quick death. I walked up to the tracks and stood there in a dazed state, listening to the approaching train. A tiny voice in my head whispered, "Why don't you try the car one more time before considering something this drastic?" I looked back at the car I had tried to coax back to life for the past hour. "What have I got to lose?"

Ethel, as I affectionately called her, started right up without a hitch. I winced. "I guess I'm going to have to face my life after all." I drove to the nearest Motel 6 and went to bed. Things would look brighter with some rest.

When I woke up, things did look brighter. I'm pretty good at picking myself up most of the time once I get past the pity roll. There was a strip joint, Doc's, across the parking lot from the motel. I would buy a beer there which I'd sip for hours while I shot pool. It was a great way to get to know some locals. I found Portland a very friendly place. I was particularly amazed that the men weren't lewd or inappropriate, considering the setting.

After three days at Motel 6, I had $10 left and no home. I called yet another roommate ad in the paper leaving a message on the recorder, and went over to Doc's once again to see if anybody might have a lead on a room. There weren't any roommate prospects there, so I went back to the motel. Kerry Sisk had returned my call.

I met Kerry that night. He had a cool house, with a deck, a hot tub and some woods out back. I didn't meet the other roommate, Steve Joy, for several weeks although I moved in the day after meeting Kerry. Kerry said he had to leave for the weekend, so he gave me a key and some paint. I traded my labor painting my room for my first month's rent, and my sister wired me a few hundred dollars to get on my feet. Maybe there was a God.

I was working pretty hard at trying to eat the right things and control my bulimia, but I still had binges. I didn't notice what all was in the food, but I tried to stay away from the obvious sugar items, except for ice cream. I couldn't live without it. My bulimia was now just a fact in my life. I was so deep in it that I didn't even put much energy into playing the denial game with it anymore, the "This is the last time I'll ever vomit my food" kind of thinking.

I was sitting on the deck one evening when I got the idea to do an infomercial. For those of you who don't know, an infomercial is a TV program that revolves around the sale of a product, a thirty-minute commercial actually. Mass education seemed to be the only way to break the cultural pattern of denial about sexual abuse. The idea spurred me to action.

I had changed the name of my rape prevention business from Personal Safety for Woman to SAVVY!. I wanted to put together an audio/video educational program for creating a personality and a lifestyle that was safe and empowering. I'd also teach some defensive tactics. Knowing and believing that you can defend yourself often prevents you from having to do so. When I carry myself as if I am "King of the Hill," I do not get targeted for unwanted behaviors and I delight in the pure joy of being in control of my life. The "King of the Hill" energy is not about ego, but about confidence.

I can size up a total stranger in a few seconds or moments by evaluating their energy. They too get to read my energy and if they sense that I am confident and un-afraid they are forced to consider why. Has she got a gun in her pocket? Is she a cop or an FBI agent? Why does she seem so sure of herself? That is what becoming savvy had done for my life. I now had an air of confidence about me instead of the essence of a victim.

I had developed a program for teaching savvy life skills to others that didn't require the ten years of dedica-tion it had taken me. Now I wanted to take my program national. The company slogan later became "When walk-ing through the jungle, don't act like food!" I think it per-fectly describes my prescription for safety.

I think I had seen a total of two infomercials be-fore embarking on this journey. Most infomercials are insulting to your intelligence, but a few are well done, sell great products, and turn some mind-boggling num-bers in sales.

Insomniacs are the bulk of infomercial buyers, since most infomercials air at midnight or later. Did I mention that I had a sleep disorder too? Years of ham-mering my body with toxic substances and living on cof-fee rendered me sleepless most nights. Go figure.

I started channel surfing for ideas. One night I surfed onto an infomercial that really caught my eye. The hostess of the show was a wild, almost bald woman named Susan Powter. She was bouncing around the set with un-bridled passion, telling the audience about her dramatic weight loss and selling her "Stop the Insanity" weight loss program.

I can do that, I thought. I have passion, a great program to sell, and my story will sell it. All I have to do is get the audio/video series produced, then I can convince somebody that my infomercial is worth investing in.

To get the series produced I needed some serious backing, which required a business plan. This was going to be a little more complicated than renting an empty building, turning on the lights and the heat, and teaching Tae Kwon-Do. I would need some business savvy. I set out to learn the ropes.

By calling a few production companies, I got an idea of what kind of information and services I was going to need. I telephoned, faxed and networked around the country.

I was told, for instance, that I would need a fulfillment company. I didn't know what that meant or what they did, so I picked one in my area and called them up. I told them that if they would take the time to educate me, show me their facility and work with SAVVY!, I would commit our business to their company. When I told them that Susan Powter had reportedly generated 100 million dollars in sales her first year out and that I was confident that SAVVY! would match or surpass that, no one turned me down.

My new friend Joel Gallob, who was a start-up environmental attorney, helped me with all the legalese while I enlisted some real marketing heavyweights to jump in with us.

I empowered a very savvy group of professionals to travel down this road with me. Mary Brelsford, who has a Masters degree in international marketing and business, wrote, published and marketed her own book, The House Diary, through her company Wow Wadda Company. John Pihas owns his own marketing firm in Portland and is rumored to be "The Dude" in the marketing business in the Northwest. Larry Anderson spent twenty-five years in radio and television. Darren O'Brian was the Creative Director for Fox 49, a local TV station. And the list of highly accomplished, passionate professionals went on and on.

I ended up with a beautiful business plan, more than worthy of the $2 million we were seeking to launch the direct-response campaign for the SAVVY! Safety Series. I had enlisted all these accomplished individuals to work for sweat equity. "Sweat equity" simply means working for a percentage of future profits from the business instead of payment up-front. We were confident that I could empower an investor to join us.

I had an idea one day. I decided to approach Chrysler with this proposal: "I'll put my new Neon in the infomercial and tell my folksy story about how the image of this car changed my life and you give me $2 million."

A company like Chrysler can blow through millions in television advertising in an afternoon. My infomercial would run continuously for months. Chrysler bit. I was invited to Detroit to talk to the top four marketing people in the company.

The trip to Detroit cost me $2000, which I have yet to pay off (thanks Marc, thanks Joey, thanks Frank). This trip turned out to be a bigger deal than I had imagined, but I didn't realize how big until it was over.

I held several meetings with my SAVVY! associates before leaving for Detroit. We eventually agreed that I should go alone. I had recruited each of them, one-on-one; why wouldn't I be able to handle the folks at Chrysler?

My partners had some concerns about my outfit of choice — designer jeans, a SAVVY! t-shirt and cowboy boots. My plan was to have a trademark outfit that I wore every day, everywhere. I would only need to pack three of each item to travel the country, eliminating several pieces of luggage.

I was greeted warmly by the powers-that-be at Chrysler. I had only been there for a moment, though, when the lone woman in the group made a comment to the effect of "Gee, you really put on the dog for us," meaning, I presumed, that I was underdressed.

I didn't miss a beat. I replied, "But the audience I am marketing to isn't you. They're at home, in their jeans and t-shirts. The American public is going to love me just the way I am." To her credit, she acknowledged my point with "You're absolutely right."

They gave me a lot of strokes on the business plan. We batted back and forth a little on the numbers, but it was just for sport — the money wasn't the issue, liability was. If anybody who purchased the series got hurt for any reason, they would be looking for the deepest pocket — Chrysler. They had already had an unpleasant experience with funding a project and then getting sued over an injury. The folks at Chrysler passed on my project but were genuinely supportive of my mission.

I could have been devastated but I wasn't. It was a real high. After all the years of being oppressed by my father, I had bellied up to the conference table, in jeans and a t-shirt, and held my own with a room full of top-ranking executives for a Fortune 50 company. I got a chunk of my power back that day that I had given away to my father years ago. Besides, they were right. The liability was a concern. If it hadn't been, I believe they would have gone for it. They claimed that they believed in my ability to succeed and invited me to keep them updated on our progress.

It was worth $2000 and a weekend of rain in the Detroit ghetto in a Super 8 Motel. There was plenty of room for optimism. We just had to look for ways to curb the liability. Tweak it a little, as they say.

After some tweaking, I took out an ad in The Wall Street Journal seeking an investor. I got calls continually for days, even months, and built a list of five respondents on the East Coast. I told each one that I was headed east to meet with the others and asked if they would like to be on my itinerary. After sitting down with each of these companies and individuals, I planned to head to Washington, D.C., for a few days for some networking there on the way home.

I thought I was so clever with my little squeeze play, leading each party to think that I had other brokers or investors vying for my attention. The joke was on me, however. Shortly after arriving, I discovered that three of them were brokers for the same venture capital giant but spread out throughout New England. Only one of them could represent SAVVY! Two names had just fallen off my list. And the venture capital company they all worked for wanted money up-front, so that eliminated all three of them anyway.

One of the investors on the list was to work with me over the phone for many months, trying to work out a deal that would serve us both. The other investor backed out at the last minute. I left New England empty-handed and headed for Washington, D.C. A friend of mine from Portland was going to be in town at the same time. We agreed to meet for a drink.

Dick and I met at Mr. Smith's, a popular D.C. piano bar named after the movie, Mr. Smith Goes to Washington. We were singing our brains out at the piano bar and swapping stories. He topped all mine with this dandy.

Although he wore an expensive suit and a Rolex, like many businessmen, Dick rarely carried any cash on him. One day he had a grand total of $2 in his pocket. Before he knew it he was surrounded by five thugs with clubs and pipes. They asked for his money, so he handed them the contents of his pockets. They were none too pleased.

One of them spotted his Rolex and barked. "We'll take that."

Dick said, "No!"

"Whadda ya mean, no?" the guy asked in amazement. "There's five of us with weapons."

Dick responded with, "Well I'm either going to take a beating now or when I get home and tell my wife that the watch she bought me is gone. I'll take my chances now." They left without the watch. Way to go, Dick!

I poured myself off the stool and headed for the bathroom after that one. On the way I ran into a very distinguished foreign-looking gentleman. He was right in my path, so I stopped to chat with him. He told me that he was the Ambassador of Bangladesh. Although he regaled me with political stories about his work for Bangladesh, I politely dismissed myself. I really had to pee.

A while later I headed to the bathroom again. Once again this well-dressed, Ghandi-looking guy was in my path. He got my attention again. After listening to him for a few more minutes, I finally stopped him and said, "You must be somebody important, everybody around here is kissing your ass and you're not tipping any of them." He roared, another guy at the top, hungry for somebody who would treat him as a peer. We became fast friends.

A few hours later, Dick and I were invited to his home, which was covered in pictures of the ambassador with celebrities and presidents. I was invited back again, alone, a few days later. Ambassador Humayan Kabir became one of my dearest friends. He agreed to deliver a letter for me about my mission to Hilary Clinton, through a mutual friend of theirs. I stayed up all night writing that letter.

I was invited back to Humayan's home for a homemade Bangladeshi meal. Humayan and I ate, drank and chatted all evening. I also got to meet one of his daughters, a sweet girl. At first he was quite naïve about the prevalence of sexual abuse; he thought I was exaggerating. I finally showed him enough evidence that he dropped his denial. He was truly overwhelmed and became the best advocate the SAVVY! company ever had.

He called me a few days after I flew back to Portland from D.C. He said he was headed to New York the following week and would try to get me in to see Barbara Walters, with whom he apparently had a friendship. I agreed to meet him in New York. I borrowed more money and got on another plane.

Barbara flew out for a Kuwaiti crisis while I was flying in. The ambassador was a kick to party with, though, so I wasn't disappointed for long. Talk about a networking fool. He came home every night with ten of the most powerful business cards in the city in his pocket.

One night we partied at Fredrick's, one of the places to be seen in Manhattan. Fredrick came out and greeted Humayan personally, and we took some pictures with him and his staff — all gorgeous, personable folks. The next night when we went back to Fredrick's, the security guard at the door wasn't going to let us in. He said it was too crowded already.

I turned to Humayan and noted loudly, "Well, gee, Ambassador, they're not going to let you in. Where would like to go instead?"

Before he could respond, the security guard threw open the doors, and parted the crowd like the Red Sea. We were escorted to the bar and offered a drink. In all my years of bar hopping I'd never thought of that line to get me in the door! Who knew?

For the next two years Humayan kept in touch with me from all over the country. "Hi, Denise, I'm here in Iowa with Jimmy Carter" or "Would you please say hi to my dear friend Senator So-and-So?" or "I'm here in

Boston with Joe Blow who owns an investment banking company." I spoke with all his high-powered friends and he spoke to anyone I asked him to say a kind word to. Everybody felt blessed to get to talk to the ambassador — he is special!

SAVVY! still had no funding so I decided to scrap and reorder. We rewrote the whole project specifically for children. They are at the most risk and a welcome marketing tool. It seemed like a natural.

I dreamed of the SAVVY! Survival Kit. I had collected some of the top children's experts in the world in personal safety. They all had great products on the market and they were all up against the same denial. The Survival Kit would come in an earth-friendly SAVVY! totebag, with a video tape that I would produce on savvy skills for kids, a safety coloring book, an illustrated book on appropriate touch, an audio sing-a-long tape, a SAVVY! t-shirt, and a bumper sticker.

The coloring book was designed by Marcia Morgan of Migima Designs. She is an ex-Portland police officer who designed the anatomical dolls that police departments use to interview young abuse victims.

The book, A Very Touching Book, was written by Jan Hindman, founder of the It's About Childhood Foundation. The book teaches children about appropriate touch with great text and darling illustrations.

The audiotape, Can't Fool Me, was produced by the Safety Child company, out of Austin, Texas. It was the hottest thing going! The disc jockey was a dinosaur who sounded like Wolfman Jack teaching safety. (800 YELLOW DINO)

We spent weeks and several more thousand dollars putting together a proposal for the Disney Company. It was awesome. We made Timone and Pumba (one very savvy character and his sidekick from The Lion King) our safety instructors. We could plug into all of Disney's resources with our slogan "When walking through the jungle, don't act like food!" It was a perfect fit.

Everybody at Disney who saw it liked it; some loved it. But I couldn't get it to the visionaries. Disney won't look at outside proposals because they are concerned about being accused of stealing properties. I kept dead-ending at the legal department.

I could tell you SAVVY! stories forever, but I'm sure my publisher would prefer that I add that topic to my future books list and move on. Suffice it to say, SAVVY! hasn't gotten its investment. The SAVVY! Safety Series concept will probably stay dusty on the shelf, but the Disney project for kids won't. I'm not through knocking on Michael Eisner's door yet.

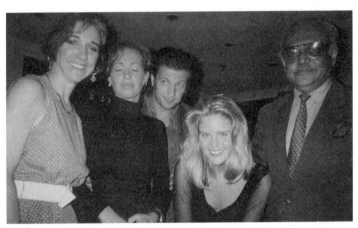

Me and the ambassador with Frederick and staff at his club in Manhattan.

Food for Thought...

Entrepreneurs are an interesting breed. And venture capital is a fascinating arena. Tenacity and perseverance are the name of the game. Smart investors don't invest in widgets or ideas. They invest in people who won't let anything get in the way of their passion. My SAVVY! experiences prepared me for my next career move. This time I only had to move about two miles as the crow flies to change my life more drastically than coming 3000 miles in the past ten years had. I didn't change venues this time. I changed dimensions.

Just for Fun...

Creativity in hunting venture capital is very important. I developed a number of techniques during my SAVVY! run for getting the attention of rich, powerful and very busy people. One of my favorites was playing fax.

I had been talking to a venture capitalist named Jeff Janda. Jeff indicated that he was interested in SAVVY! and that he would get back to me. He was such a busy man, though, that it was hard to get his attention. One day when I spoke with him he told me that he had been off at some big-shot gig doing a promotion for my nemesis, Farrah Fawcett.

A few weeks later, when I still hadn't gotten a response from Jeff, I faxed him a letter that read:

"I started out with nothing and I still have half of it left, but it's going to be all gone if you don't move on my project soon. I may not be as famous as Farrah, but I will be if you bankroll my company!" Jeff called me five minutes later.

Out on a Limb

I should back up a little. For the last year and a half of my run with SAVVY! I was living with an old man named Fred. Kerry had sold his wonderful house after I'd lived there just a few months, but Fred's was even nicer. It sat on 1.3 acres in a quaint old neighborhood that he had helped to pioneer. I had the whole downstairs of the house to myself. There was a waterbed in my oversized room, a big Jacuzzi in my bathroom, a fireplace in the den I used for my office and a washer and dryer right down the hall.

Fred was so lonely when I met him that he all but begged me to move in with him. He was sixty-nine to my thirty-seven and our birthdays were three days apart. He offered me free rent for six months to help me get my company off the ground. After that he charged me $300 a month. It was a great deal — most days.

Fred and I had a volatile love/hate friendship. The problem was that he was in love with me and he refused to let go of the notion that I would someday jump in bed with him and fulfill his fantasies. I happen to love old men. If he had been a harmless old coot it wouldn't have been a problem, but he wasn't.

Fred made lewd or demeaning comments way too often to get along with me. I would rage at him, but he wouldn't stop his behaviors. I would talk to him about it rationally when I wasn't seething mad over his latest sexist remark. I'd say, "Fred, I'm your closest friend in the world right now, and I know that in many ways you really respect me, so why would you continually say offensive things to me? You would never treat any of your other friends this way."

He'd think for a moment and respond, "I don't know."

Once I was so offended by one of his "Hey, baby, nice tits" comments that I warned, "Fred, I would hate to have to get violent with an old man, but if you ever say something like that to me again I am going to kick you!" Fred liked to play the macho role but he was genuinely intimidated by my martial arts skills.

A few days later, Joel (my attorney friend) came over to work on some contracts for SAVVY!. Fred came down to my room for something and made one of his unwelcome comments. I picked up my leg and kicked his protruding belly. I didn't hit him very hard, but I did it so fast that it frightened him. He turned to Joel and started whining that I had tried to kill him. From then on he was sincerely afraid of me but still couldn't hold his tongue.

The upside was that we had some great times. We'd watch Jeopardy and Wheel of Fortune together most evenings, then trade stories. I would tell him the latest SAVVY! antics and he would tell me the same tales from the "good old days" over and over and over. And Fred loved to hear me practice the piano. I spent three months working on my own arrangement of "Frosty the Snowman" and Fred loved every horrible rendering.

The phone and the fax were humming all the time and SAVVY! associates frequently dropped by. Fred would try to engage them in conversation as they headed down the stairs to my space, but they all knew better. To keep you in the room, Fred could tell a thirty-minute story without taking a breath. The only person who could out-talk him was Lowell.

I'd come home and Fred would be bitching and rolling his eyes, complaining that Lowell had called and talked his face off in my absence. I'd note, "Well, next time you see that 'I'm going to pass out if you don't take a breath' look on my face, you'll know what it means!"

Fred had diabetes. He had been diagnosed twelve years before. He was a pro at controlling his diabetes with diet and didn't need insulin at all if he ate well. The diabetes had made him impotent, though, which I suspect generated much of the shame that caused Fred to be so sexually offensive.

Interesting manifestation for me, wouldn't you say? I end up living with a man old enough to be my father, with whom I have a love/hate relationship, who is sexually offensive towards me, and who is surviving a degenerative disease only because of his diet — my life's issues all wrapped up in one semi-vertical, wrinkled pile.

Only one of Fred's six children was speaking to him when I moved in, and his ex-wife had taken him for quite a ride. He was a bitter man. The only thing that he truly loved was his gardening. He loved to plant and tinker with the landscaping. He also loved his fruit trees.

After a year and a half, the friction between Fred and me became too much. Fred asked me to move out. He had talked himself into believing that if I moved out, his son, who lived a few miles away, would move in. Apparently, his son was unaware of this.

I told almost all my friends and associates, "You just watch. Fred will be dead within two months after I move out." I believed this because I had watched Fred's diabetes rise and fall with his depression, which was determined by how well he ate. When I was around, spending time with him and stroking his ego, he ate great, felt great, and needed no insulin. When I was busy and unavailable, or pissed and unfriendly, he turned to sweets, and his depression and his diabetes kicked his ass.

I ended up moving in with an acquaintance and her precious daughter, Maggie. Dorothy Cole had a Masters in Education and a lot of experience as an entrepreneur. Maggie, who was nine at the time, was one exceptional kid.

Their house was only two miles as the crow flies from Fred's, but it felt like another planet. What a treat to be living with females who were fun and supportive. How nice to bend over the trash can and not hear some crude comment about my ass.

It was also the first time I had ever shared a space with cats — interesting beings. I had harbored a disdain for cats, not having experienced them, because my father felt that felines were only useful for target shooting.

We all have a particular method for changing gears in our lives. Some people benefit from a kick in the butt, others need a building dropped on them. Dorothy preferred car accidents. She humbly admits that she often needs a good thump on the head for the Universe to get her attention. I believe the figure was ten accidents over twenty years.

The Universe must have had some really big news for Dorothy, for the last bump on the head put her down hard. She sustained a closed head injury that sent her to bed for a year and a half and opened up a whole new facet of her life. As a result of this latest accident, she came to believe she had a gift for healing with her hands.

I was in pain almost constantly by the time I got to Dorothy's. So, I decided to let Dorothy lay her hands on me. When she did they would be burning hot. I could feel the energy run through my body.

I always got some short-term relief, but her efforts didn't cure me. My personal belief is that we have to take responsibility for why we are sick and address the cause rather than tend to the symptoms. I knew I would have to beat my eating disorder to turn my health around. But living with Dorothy and Maggie was a life-altering experience anyway. Because of what was happening with her hands, Dorothy had embarked on a spiritual awakening. She had been academically trained, but she couldn't deny that some very unscientific things were happening to her. She read all the top cult books on spirituality and paranormal phenomena. She meditated daily and became connected to some well-respected channelers and psychics.

I made another expensive attempt at teaching some rape prevention classes. I put out five hundred beautiful multicolored flyers, had a local newspaper do a feature story on me, rented conference rooms, and spent weeks networking with related agencies. Not one person showed up for my classes. I was pretty worn out with the whole business but didn't know what to do.

So, I did what many people do when they get over-whelmed by their life: I got sick. As I recall, it was the achy joints, headache and fever, the "I just want to die" thing. I would obviously be spending a few days hanging around the house, so Dorothy pulled out her video recording of Out On A Limb for me to watch.

Shirley MacLaine had starred in this four-day television miniseries that was taken from her book of the same title. I think it came out in the mid-seventies (I'm terrible with dates). It is Shirley's autobiographical account of her spiritual awakening. I imagine that she got crucified for it. She was way ahead of her time. This movie changed my life forever. Thanks, Shirley! Run it again, the time is right.

I believe the reason that Shirley's story touched me so deeply is that she was rich, famous and skinny, all the things that I thought would heal my life. Yet she still felt something was missing from hers. She wasn't complaining, mind you. She is very grateful for all the success and abundance she has been blessed with. But she still felt a void, as if she wasn't quite whole. What she was missing, she realized, was a personal relationship with God.

Shirley's spiritual awakening had taken her on a wild trip through the Andes of Peru, where she had some extraordinary other-dimensional experiences. I would watch all four hours of the series, rewind it, and start it again. It spurred something in me; it felt familiar. I almost felt as if I had lived it myself. Most of all, I believed it, which meant I had to rethink everything else that I believed.

Dorothy also turned me on to Shirley MacLaine's Inner Workout video. The tape was a result of the information that Ms. MacLaine received in Peru and felt obligated to share. It teaches us about the subtle energy systems in our bodies and how to work with them. It helped me get to places in myself that I had never reached before. I was "feeling" again. Unfortunately, most of what I was feeling was emptiness, loss and confusion.

I had been mad at God for so long that I had a lot of work to do to heal my own relationship with Spirit. And after Out On A Limb, I had to decide what I thought God was and how it fit into my life.

A few days later I went to an event at a New Age gathering place that brought in all types of speakers, healers and music. This particular evening they were sponsoring a didgeridoo player from Seattle named Carl Sacksteber. The didgeridoo is a hollowed-out tube that the Aborigines use for communication and healing. Some are made from bamboo, others from cactus. Carl even had a few that he had fashioned from PVC pipe.

Didgeridoos are magical-looking instruments and the sound (drone) that comes out of them goes right through you. It is a form of vibrational therapy. After the concert Carl promised to "didg" each one of us — playing the instrument directly over our bodies. He believed this activated the chakras (energy pathways of the body), like acupuncture without the needles.

I could feel the vibrations as Carl didged the people around me. I was sitting cross-legged on the floor when he walked up to me, pointed this wild-looking thing at my abdomen, and blew a drone. In a millisecond I experienced the most sexual moment I have ever known in my life. I looked up at this man in shock, but I had a sense that it had nothing to do with him. It was over in a second and I relaxed and enjoyed the rest of my didg. Carl played the digeridoo a few inches from my body for about three minutes, never actually touching me. There were about twenty other people that got didged that night. Everybody was moved by this experience. I was in a strange trance-like state when I left there.

The next morning my breasts were swollen, my abdomen was bloated, I was nauseous, and had to pee every few minutes. I felt pregnant, but hadn't had sex in months, and I was still in a strange mental fog.

The following evening I was at Joel's working on more SAVVY! stuff, still feeling dazed. We were sitting on the floor and I was staring up at the corner of the ceiling. I could hear Joel talking but it was as if he were miles away. I felt drugged. I then felt something lift out of my body. I could actually see this "energy" floating away from me. A moment later the spell broke and the daze lifted. I felt that I was back, and all my pregnant symptoms went away in a matter of hours. I told Joel what I had just experienced. He looked overwhelmed and his expression told me that he thought I was crazy, too.

I decided that I would tell Dorothy about this experience, but was a bit afraid she might think I was a nut case and throw me out. I gingerly led into my story. She piped up right away, "Oh, yeah, you had a psychic pregnancy. I've had several. It is a phenomenon that lots of women claim to have experienced." I didn't know what to do with that statement.

When Carl (the didgeridoo player) came back to town I invited him to stay at our house. One night he taught me how to play the didgeridoo and then went off to bed. By the time he got up the next morning I had been to the plumbing supply store and bought $50 worth of PVC connecting pieces and spray paint. I had turned the living room into a didgeridoo factory. Carl loved it — a fellow addict!

Eventually I purchased an authentic didgeridoo and hauled it with me everywhere, including board meetings, bars and restaurants. Although I didn't play that well, it doesn't take much to be able to didg other people, a simple drone will do. I had gone from being "The Karate Lady" to "The SAVVY! Lady" to "The Didgeridoo Lady." Anyone who knew me intimately thought I was crazy anyway, so it really didn't change things much.

Dorothy had a friend who was a renowned psychic – Badeish Lange. She agreed to trade me a reading for a didg. Badeish told me a lot of interesting things about my life during that reading. She seemed to think that I was on the threshold of a new beginning. I hoped she was right.

Her husband, John Paul, owned an art gallery, which splashed over into their home. Their living room was covered with beautiful works and artifacts, a very inspiring room. Badeish led me to her magical living room for her didg. She sat upright in a chair and took a couple of deep breaths with her eyes closed.

I started to play over her. I could tell immediately that she had left her body. She had that "out to lunch" look on her face, even though her eyes were closed. I was a little concerned about overwhelming her, as she was so sensitive, being a psychic.

I stopped to ask her if she was okay. She didn't answer. She struggled to open her eyes. I asked her again if she was okay. Badeish sat perfectly still, like a statue. A single tear rolled down her cheek.

Eventually she came around. She told me a vivid story about the inner voyage she had just embarked on. The story was laced with colors, lots of gold and symbols. At the end of her vision she was lying on a table surrounded by beings playing the didgeridoo. She noted that she was told to tell me that I am an extraterrestrial and that the didgeridoo is very important.

I accepted the news as a matter of fact. Everything that Badeish had told me thus far had been true or come true and she had a thriving practice of people who sought her guidance.

When I got back to Dorothy's I fell apart. "What the hell is going on?" I cried. Dorothy laughed, sat down beside me and gave me a hug. All of this seemed quite normal to her, as she had been studying all this "wu wu" stuff since her latest accident. It wasn't that I didn't believe any of it. I just didn't know what to do with all the information I had received. As a result of the Girl Scout séance incident, though, I was more prepared for looking at such things, but still very confused about my beliefs.

When I was in Las Vegas I had had an out-of-body experience just like the one Shirley MacLaine takes us on in Out On A Limb. Watching the movie and seeing that someone else had experienced exactly the same thing was astounding. I set out to read some books, meditate and search for my beliefs. I was trying to make up with God, but since I didn't know what I now believed, I didn't know how to fix that relationship.

Maggie and I would often jump in my car and head to 7-Eleven for our candy fix. Dorothy finally raged at me one day and told me to stop filling her daughter full of candy. Maggie was on homeopathic remedies for her Attention Deficit Disorder and sugar was a major no-no. I agreed to stop doing that, but it wasn't easy. Like many adults, I had used candy as a way of bonding with this kid. It is a lot more work to have a friendship with a child that revolves around activities and conversation than one that revolves around handing out forbidden treats.

I had only called Fred a couple of times since I had moved out. He sounded pretty depressed when I spoke with him and each time he said, "I think Allen is moving in next week."

This time when I called, one of his other sons answered the phone. Fred was in the hospital. He had gone in to have a toe amputated because his diabetes had worsened. He'd had a stroke on the operating table. They were going to be moving him to a hospice that day. Fred did not want to be kept alive. He had made that clear to everyone and had gotten it in the appropriate legalese. It was a little under two months since I had moved out.

I went to visit Fred in the hospice. His left side was paralyzed. He could barely move and couldn't speak at all, but it was obvious to me from the start that he was "in there."

I still had a lot of anger at this man, but I decided that I would put it aside and be there for him on his deathbed. I was doing it for my own healing and experience, not out of obligation to a dying man. I don't think that dying changes anything. It doesn't heal all wounds or require that everyone automatically forgive the deceased. It is a process that we all must go through. I was curious and saw an opportunity to go through it with Fred.

I stayed with Fred for ten hours that day. I sat and sometimes lay on the bed with him and talked and stroked his head. I told jokes and poked fun at him. I could feel that he was genuinely grateful that I had come. I said, "Well, buddy, you finally got me in bed. It only cost you a toe, your speech and probably your life. Was it worth it?" I could see a faint wrinkle by his eyes. He was trying to laugh.

At one point I was quite blunt with him. "You know, Fred, you are forced to look at the idea that karma exists, and that what you put out came back to haunt you. How many times did I ask you to stop saying offensive things to me, but you wouldn't? Now here we are, you're dying and you can't speak, and I get the last word. I forgive you, Fred, and I thank you for everything you did for me. I wish you peace." It was a very healing moment for me. I sensed that it was for Fred as well.

The nurse came to dress Fred's leg. After amputating his toe they'd had to dig a trench up his leg to drain the gangrene; it was gross. I was sitting on the bed next to Fred while she was working on his leg.

"What do you do when the patient dies?" I inquired. I had heard they had a lovely ceremony, sang and lit candles and such.

The nurse's eyes bugged out and she nodded towards Fred as if to say, "But he'll hear me!"

I responded with, "Well, he's the one dying, I'm sure he'd like to know." She rattled off the details of the touching ritual that the family and staff participated in after the patient passes. I turned to Fred and said, "Gee, Fred, what a great place you picked to die in. That sounds wonderful!"

The next day I brought Dorothy back with me to see Fred. She had been doing work with families who had lost loved ones. She had gained a reputation as one who could speak to beings on the "other side." Perhaps she could communicate with Fred or at least talk to him openly about passing over.

I was sitting on the bed next to Fred and Dorothy was sitting on the windowsill. As I talked to Fred, I saw him look around me and try to get Dorothy's attention.

She said, "He wants to know if Ruth is going to be there when he gets there." Ruth was Fred's first wife who had died of cancer. He missed her dearly.

"Of course she'll be there, Fred," I assured him. "She's waiting for you." I placed a rose on his chest. "Take this to her."

Dorothy spoke again. "He wants you to know that he really loves you and appreciates the fact that you came to see him."

I patted his hand. "I know that, Fred. I know that you would have done the same for me."

"He wants to know if Ruth will have angel wings when he sees her."

I laughed, "How the hell would I know? But I want a full report when you get there. Call Dorothy or something."

Just then Fred's daughter started to come in the room. I asked her to wait outside for a moment, which didn't go over well as she had driven a long way. We quickly said good-bye to Fred and left.

Just for the record, knowing Fred as intimately as I did, I can tell you that the conversation that transpired through Dorothy seemed real to me. Everything she said sounded like something I believed Fred would ask or say.

A few days later, after spending the evening with all his children, Fred passed on. They lit candles, sang, held hands and said good-bye. In some ways I was relieved, yet I had some guilt and regret. I felt responsible because I had known it would happen. I should have done more, but I just couldn't handle him anymore by the time I had moved out.

A week or so later, Dorothy was having a massage in her bedroom when Kiara, her massage therapist, called me in. Dorothy said, "Fred is here. My left side is numb and I can feel him in my aura." I believed her. She went on, "He wants you to contact Cindy and tell her that he's sorry." Cindy was the daughter whom I had met briefly at the hospice.

I started shaking my head no. "I don't want anything to do with that. Most of his family isn't speaking to me and I don't even know this woman. No way! I am not taking responsibility for that information." I left the room. A few days later it happened again. Dorothy called me into her room. This time she said, "Fred's back, and it's really uncomfortable having him in my aura, so I'd like for you two to work this out."

"Okay." I agreed. "What does he want?"

She repeated, "He wants you to contact Cindy and tell her he's sorry." Reluctantly, I said I would do so when the time was right.

For some reason I had a ton of anxiety about making this phone call. I kept putting it off and putting it off until it finally fell out of my consciousness. (New age jargon for "I forgot about it.") And, of course, I lost her number. It wasn't until a year and a half later that I called Fred's son Rick and asked him to tell Cindy. He felt I should be the one to explain it to her.

I went on another anxiety roll for a couple of weeks before I finally found the courage to call her. Let's face it, this is a pretty wild story to tell a perfect stranger. I introduced myself and led into my tale. She was quiet as I unfolded it. When I finished I nervously paused, and she began to speak.

"It's amazing that you would pick today to call me! I had the strangest experience in art therapy class today. I had this wonderful feeling wash over me, and for the first time in my life, I'm at peace with my father. And then you call and tell me this story. What a wonderful gift," she said sweetly.

We talked for quite some time and I really felt a bond with her. I haven't spoken to her since, but I have a warm spot in my heart for Cindy. What a touching closure between Fred and Cindy, and I got to be the messenger.

I went to see Badeish again. I loved the way she glowed when her husband was around. John Paul was a model partner, and they were crazy in love and truly genuine, interesting and fun to be around. This particular day I said to her, "I want what you have. I want a relationship like yours." She told me a delightful story of how John Paul had magically come into her life after she had said a certain prayer. She had also done a lot of emotional work beforehand. She did a guided meditation with me and showed me how to say the prayer and visualize the kind of mate I wanted to find. I lit a candle and some incense that night and stared at the stars through the window while I lay in bed and said that prayer.

The following week Dorothy held her usual Saturday night meditation group. An interesting fellow showed up that night with a young friend. Patrick was six-foot-three and at the time he had long hair, a full beard, intense big eyes and talked a lot. Pat was an organic worm farmer and spoke, ad nausem, about the need to build gardens, build up the soil and heal the food supply.

Suffice it to say, Patrick McEachern turned out to be my next prince, and he had just waltzed in the front door.

Before long I moved another two miles to Pat's organic farm and stepped into yet another dimension. James Redfield, author of The Celestine Prophecy, would be moved by this place. It was better than Oz.

FOOD FOR THOUGHT...

It doesn't matter how much of this chapter you can, or choose, to believe. It was real to me and drove me to reevaluate my entire way of looking at life.

The search for my spiritual beliefs was scary, but a lot more fun than the search for my memories had been. I often had to trust my feelings instead of my intellect. In time I forged a belief system that works for me.

I cherish the memories of Fred and the hospice. Those were really tender moments for Fred and me, a connection we couldn't seem to muster until he was dying.

To me, death doesn't have to be a horrifying experience. When we can let go of the fear and face it with awe and curiosity, I believe it makes the journey that much richer for all concerned.

JUST FOR FUN...

I swear to God, I found the following quip about a man named Fred. Fred would have loved this joke.

Fred was in the hospital, near death, so the family sent for his pastor. As the pastor stood beside the bed, Fred's frail condition grew worse. He motioned frantically for something to write on. The pastor lovingly handed him a pen and a piece of paper. Fred used his last ounce of strength to scribble a note, then died. The pastor thought it best not to look at the note just then, so he slipped it into his jacket pocket.

At the funeral several days later the pastor delivered the eulogy. He realized he was wearing the same jacket that he'd worn the day that Fred had died.

"You know," he said, "Fred handed me a note just before he died. I haven't read it, but knowing Fred, I'm sure there's a word of inspiration there for us all." He unfolded the note and read aloud:

"You're standing on my oxygen tube!"

The Edge, The Oregonian, Portland, Oregon 12/3/1997

THE MAGIC GARDEN

When I was nine my sister handed me a book that touched me deeply. It was a true story about a community of people in Findhorn, Scotland. They worked with the nature spirits to grow magical produce, gently tilling the soil by hand and planting their loving intention with every seed. They graced The Guinness Book of World Records for growing lettuce the size of Volkswagens and tomatoes that barely fit in wheelbarrows. I wanted to go there so bad.

Twenty-seven years after reading The Magic of Findhorn, I moved onto an organic farm with Pat and his delightful twelve-year-old son, Patrick. Pat farmed worms, danced with the devas (nature spirits) and talked to trees. The farm was everything I had dreamed it would be.

This little patch of "Findhorn" had started out a barren field on the edge of a forest. With the help of his brother, Mike, and friends Bob and Christian, Pat had built a four-directional Hopi Indian garden, and a fire pit in the woods surrounded by hand-hewn chairs made from tree stumps.

Pat and his former wife, Betty, had created a labyrinth. Its pathways were lined with cobblestones and river rocks. They constructed bridges over the streams that flowed through this natural wetlands and hauled in fifty-six dump trucks full of the finest topsoil nature could produce from a neighboring worm farm.

The fruit trees and grapevines they planted brought in the birds en masse. Deer came through this wooded corridor on their way up the mountain, and red-tailed hawks hovered overhead in reverence of this very special place.

At times the frogs would croak us a symphony at daybreak, accompanied by a choir of mourning doves. Pat's farm was better than Findhorn; it was more magical than Oz. It was Heaven!

My favorite part of living on the farm was the animals. Animals are great healing tools, especially for those of us who have trouble bonding with humans. For children, our furry friends are a powerful elixir.

We had two chickens, briefly — the dogs ate them. We had a rabbit that I named Theodore, but he died. And there was Butterscotch, a sweet calico cat. She was so elusive that I didn't even know she lived on the farm for the first six months. Eventually she gifted us with fourteen delightful cats.

First there was the litter with Sam, Dan and Bob. They each eventually fathered a litter with Butterscotch. They all turned out to be devoted mates to her in turn, and produced some lovely kitties, only one of which had any genetic challenges from the interbreeding. Out of the next litter we kept Sage, Pumpkin and Snowflake. And finally there were Maya and Frank. These little beings were like my children. They brought me more joy than anything money can buy.

Pat and Patrick had three dogs — Luie, Shadow and Scoobie. Luie was old, crippled and sick. The two young pups would trample over him mercilessly all day, trying to get our attention. Everybody loved and felt sorry for Luie, so he got the most affection. I had taken to didging Luie's ailing hips. The other dogs would run from the didgeridoo; eventually Luie came to like it.

None of the dogs were allowed in the garden. One day Luie was sunning himself near the entrance to the Hopi garden when I went out to didg him. Before long he got up and hobbled in and lay down among the flowers. This was not like Luie. Amazingly though, he had planted his large butt perfectly between the flowers without harming any of them, but I was in a panic.

I started out by talking to Luie, then yelling at him and then beating on him in an attempt to get him out of the garden. He would get up, waddle a foot and then plop down in the flowers again, each time perfectly positioned so as not to harm a single petal. I was finally overcome with guilt for beating on this old, sick dog and gave up.

When I began to didg Luie's hips, I received a very strong intuition. "Oh, he's lying down in the flowers. Luie is trying to tell me that he's dying." I cried and hugged him and didged him for a long time. After I stopped he got up and lumbered out of the garden. The next morning Pat came in crying. Luie was dead. Pat lovingly buried him in the "O" of our raised-bed garden that spelled LOVE.

Eventually Bob the turtle came to live with us. Bob was a trip. When we adopted him he lived in a tiny glass aquarium. One day Pat came in to find Bob executing an escape. He had his front hand(?), paw(?), whatever, up on the top of the aquarium. As Pat watched, Bob pulled himself up until he got his shell teetering on the edge. He then rocked himself until he fell over the side onto the floor.

After that, we decided that Bob was a rambling man and gave him free range of the house. He would cruise all over the place but we never saw him do it. We would just find him behind the dryer or the woodburning stove.

One time the phone was down all weekend. We assumed that they had shut it off because we were behind on the bill. I hadn't seen Bob for days and remembered that he liked to wedge himself between the refrigerator and the wall. That's exactly where I found him — sitting on the phone line that he had unplugged.

I finally had the horse that I had dreamed of since childhood. Sid was a very special being too. Sid's hooves were in bad shape, so we didn't ride him much. He was just a friend and supplied manure for the worms, but I really wanted to ride him bareback, just once, to see if I could do it.

I fed him, brushed him, talked to him and most of all listened to him. It took me about six months to realize that he was communicating with me. When I finally got it, it blew me away. He wasn't just saying things like "Did you bring me any oats?" He would give me insights into my emotional baggage.

One thing I distinctly remember from the Girl Scout riding camps I had attended is that horses can sense your fear. I kept asking Sid for a bareback gallop around the corral, but every time I got on his back without the saddle he would refuse to budge.

The voice I kept hearing said, "You're afraid."

I would respond, "No I'm not!"

One day I said, "Okay, Sid, I'll leave you alone, but how about a ride for my birthday? That's not too much to ask, is it? I drag myself out here at night in the freezing cold to feed you. I just want one little ride." I thought we had a deal.

I excitedly waited for my birthday believing that Sid would comply. First thing that morning I put the bridle on him and climbed onto his back. He wouldn't budge. I was disappointed and angry. I sat on his back for quite some time talking and complaining.

He kept saying (via a little voice in my head, of course), "You're afraid."

"No, I'm not!" I would defiantly bark back. Later that day I tried again, same result. After trying everything to get Sid to move I just sat on his back. Eventually my mind wandered. The moment I stopped thinking about riding him and relaxed, he took off running. I just about fell off, but managed to get balanced and enjoy the short gallop.

He stopped dead and teased, "I told you. You were afraid."

"Yup, you were right," I admitted. "But I'm not scared anymore. Thanks, Sid!"

There were some other critters on the farm that I learned to love too — the snakes.

Since early childhood I had been — I can't even think of a word vivid enough — let's say "morbidly afraid" of snakes. My sister theorized that as a child I subconsciously projected the fear I had of my father on these slithery little devils that lived out in the woods. In my first fifteen years in New York, I think I had seen a total of two snakes, so it was a fairly safe place to park my fear.

When we moved onto a golf course in Houston, where all the water holes were infested with water moccasins the size of Cadillacs, so to speak, it got a little trickier. I had nightmares about snakes that would traumatize me for days. And these continued to occur over many years.

I had worked on this fear in therapy and on my own. I had tried going to a pet store just to look at the snakes in the window and ended up either paralyzed with fear or running in terror. I couldn't seem to beat it.

A snake the size of a Cadillac is unnerving, but it can be seen from a distance and is easy to run from. But the tiny little garter snakes on Pat's farm were even scarier because they were so fast and just appeared at your feet without warning. Not to mention that they were everywhere, all summer.

I knew when I decided to move onto the farm that I was going to have to conquer this fear or live in terror. I began the process of breaking my fear by picturing them the way Gary Larson, the cartoonist who produces The Far Side, does. I would imagine the snakes with little horned-rimmed glasses and bow ties around their necks. It really helped.

Then I started to envision them as spiritual Findhorn-type beings, a necessary part of the garden. They eat certain destructive insects. That helped too.

It took me about a year, but I finally got to the point where I could pick up the snakes and talk to them. I was still anxious, but the feeling of being in control of that fear was so exhilarating that I considered them a great gift.

The labyrinth was my favorite spot on the property. A labyrinth is a circular geometrical pattern laid out on the ground, and occasionally indoors, that one walks. Some religions have spiritual beliefs about labyrinths. Many people simply consider them a nice meditative place to walk. There was definitely something special going on in this particular labyrinth.

As I mentioned, the labyrinth was lined with cobblestones and river rocks. The wildflowers would grow to shoulder height during the summer so that you were walking through a maze of flowers and scents, while the birds provided the music.

The wildlife, and the domestic animals, were also attracted to the labyrinth. Somedays we'd have to move Sid and the numerous piles he had gifted us with out first before we could traverse the pathways. The cats loved it too.

One morning I watched as a deer peered curiously over the fence at the labyrinth. It stood there for the longest time, nervously looking around until it finally found the courage to hop the fence and stand in the labyrinth. The deer stood there transfixed, apparently soaking up the feeling of standing on such sacred ground.

Romantically, Pat and I had a rough beginning. He hadn't gotten over his third wife, Betty, and was still in love with a woman who had captured his heart twenty years before. There was little room left for me.

For my part, I was more in love with what he knew than who he was. I slept with him because I wanted to be part of his Findhorn world, but I really didn't let him in. And he wanted nothing to do with my world of business and venture capital. Consequently, we were like two screaming three-year-olds trying to get our emotional needs met; it became quite a competition. That's the bad news. The good news is that we helped each other a lot.

The very first night that we slept together, Pat had put his hand on my back. His hands were even hotter and more magical than Dorothy's. I welcomed his healing energy whenever he would share it. Unfortunately, I got a lot more attention from him when I was sick. Fortunately, I was very sick.

Pat told me one day that my liver was in trouble. I remember that moment very vividly. I was sitting on the couch and he was sitting across from me. As the words came out of his mouth, this fog descended on my brain, pushing away the possibility that what he had said could be true. I now recognize that fog as denial. I just didn't want to hear what he was telling me. The symptoms I had described to him were those I had experienced since I was a teen. I didn't want to believe that my liver had been in trouble that long. I told him that he was wrong.

Two days later I rescinded that statement. "I'm sure you're right about my liver," I admitted. "I just didn't want to face the possibility that my body has been distressed that long, but I can see that denial isn't going to help."

One morning soon after, my back was in excruciating pain. I sat down and cried. I begged Pat to help me with my health. He wasn't very supportive. His attitude was "Yeah, sure. Everybody says that, but nobody really wants to do it." He had been talking to people about food and health for twenty years. Lots of people had shown some interest but disappeared when it came time to do any work in the garden or give up their favorite treats.

I assured him that I would be different. He refused to believe it.

I chuckled to myself remembering the day that I had made Yung apologize to me after outliving his "You won't last a week" prediction by ten years. "We'll just see, Pat."

I ate everything that Pat fed me and took any supplement or herb he recommended. I still had binges, though. Baskin and Robbins had my heart. I tried switching to some of the sugar-free flavors, but then usually had them load a pile of fudge ripple on top. What's the point of a binge if you are going to eliminate the decadent items you're not supposed to have! Besides, if you're not planning on keeping it down, what's the difference?

I noticed that it was always refined carbohydrates that set off my binges — sugar. Even foods like organic pretzels turn into sugar in the blood stream, launching the blood-sugar roller-coaster. For those of us who love the rush of our pancreas scrambling to keep us alive, there's nothing like sugar!

I was dedicated to giving up cigarettes. I had been banished outside to smoke, which slowed me down a little. Every time Pat said something about my smoking, I would admit, "I know they're poison. I'm really trying to quit, but I'm so anxious right now."

Pat was very supportive of that. He knew how wickedly addictive cigarettes are. He had taken up smoking, although very lightly, when Betty and he had lived together and even he had had a hell of a time kicking the habit.

It took me four months to beat the cigarettes altogether. After that, when I would bum the occasional puff off somebody, I'd gag. How had I ever put these disgusting things in my mouth for so long?

My health improved slowly. My back was definitely improving as my diet did. I continued to get my share of acne, though, which I picked at obsessively, another of the dysfunctions I had carried with me from puberty. But I was beginning to recognize that the acne was directly linked to my eating habits and hydration. The better I ate, and the more pure water I drank, the better my skin was.

Pat and I were living hand to mouth most of the time. We would do a landscaping, concrete or remodeling job, and then work the farm until the money ran out. One time when the money ran out we couldn't find work right away. We didn't have five dollars to go into town to buy anything, and the cupboards were bare. All we had to eat was a little bit of produce plucked out of the garden, but it was energized, mineralized, fresh food. When what we ate was limited to only that, we changed, forever!

It was like Dorothy landing in Oz. We hadn't plopped our house down on a witch, but we had certainly landed in another dimension. It was also like flying — when you take off in lousy weather and then ascend above the clouds and see the sunshine. The fog had lifted, and I saw myself, my life, and God in a whole new magnificent light.

This is what I mean by "Eating My Way to Heaven." And for the first time in my life, through this magical food, I experienced the feeling of unconditional love. It was a pervasive, all-encompassing love. Pat felt it too.

God, Great Spirit, The Universal Consciousness — whatever you want to call it — was speaking to me, and for the first time in twenty years, I was listening. It was as if I had been living in a foreign land all my life and finally learned to understand the language.

Out of this new clarity of perception came a constant rush of information. Every bird that flew by, every billboard I saw, every commercial on TV appeared to be a symbol of some sort, and I knew what each one meant.

Another thing that occurred from eating nothing but the food in the magic garden was that my senses became very acute. One day I was walking the labyrinth and Shadow was about fifty feet away stalking a field mouse. I stopped to watch him. He had his front leg raised and bent as he intently observed his prey. He then took a step forward in slow motion. As he placed his front paw on the ground I heard the crunch of a blade of grass. Then I thought, "Wait a minute. The dog is fifty feet away from me, tiptoeing through the field, and I heard a blade of grass crunch. That's impossible!"

Shadow methodically took another step. I heard another crunch. I pondered, "Either I am hallucinating, or I have received a wonderful gift."

Pat and Joel and I were walking the labyrinth together close to dusk one afternoon during this period of sacred eating. The guys were a ways behind me when I stopped dead in my tracks. The plants were doing a 3-D dance for me. One leaf would jump up in my face and catch my attention and then descend into the background, as another leaf would jump up at me. I stood there in awe thinking, "Gee, I spent a fortune on drugs in my lifetime and never saw anything like this. Wow!"

Wow, is right. Who knew that our bodies were intended to be conduits for Spirit, and that if we would just stop poisoning them and feed them what God gives us to eat, God's voice would be loud and clear. Pat and I now knew this, but that didn't mean we could live it all the time.

That was the experience I had been searching for since reading The Magic of Findhorn in childhood — reveling in unconditional love, and glowing and dancing with the devas. I thought that once I found that gateway to heaven I would never turn back. It hasn't been that easy.

We were still addicted to refined treats, even though the ones we chose were healthier than most. We still liked our organic pretzels and chips and goodies, and we were occasionally eating breads with sugar and consuming honey and maple syrup. Only whole foods have that consciousness-altering life force. Honey and maple syrup in their natural form have nutrients that are helpful, but as with all forms of sugar, it's hard not to do too much. The consumption of these foods brought us right back down to earth.

Whole foods, (we affectionately call them suPRANAtural™ foods) are ones that come straight off the tree, vine or bush, which is growing in energized soil that has been built up and mineralized. Worm castings (polite name for worm droppings) add the essential microorganisms to the soil, and ultimately our food, that aids us in digesting it.

Crops grown in dead soil that has been chemically farmed may look whole and nutritious, but it is just an illusion. They are void of balanced nutrition and that consciousness-raising life force that transformed me, not to mention all the toxic substances they do contain, like herbicides, pesticides and fertilizers.

Pat had learned how to farm worms from his friend Bob Buss. Like many ex-pot growers, Bob had learned the value of rich soil. In the marijuana industry the difference between a good plant and a great one was thousands of dollars. Looks don't count much — it's the quality of the plant that brings a good return. It was worth his time to learn how to build up the soil. Nobody knew how to make the worms dance like Bob the Worm Man. He considered the worms his friends.

Cleopatra and Darwin were also savvy about worms. Cleopatra considered them sacred animals. Removal of worms from any of her territories was punishable by death. Darwin called them the guts of the soil. And in a litigation that Bob was involved in, worms were deemed livestock in Oregon and protected under the same laws.

Our friends and family members thought that we had gone over the edge. We knew we had definitely crossed over a line and there would be no going back. Back up a tidge now and then, yes. Go back, never! Pat and I made a deeper commitment to spread the word about food and health and God.

I heard a speaker at the Living Enrichment Center pull out that age old quote from Jesus that so many people use to justify their eating habits.

"Take no thought for your life, for what you shall eat." (Luke 12:22)

First of all there were no Twinkies and Cokes 2000 years ago. Secondly, I don't believe that Jesus was trying to say, "Just eat any old thing." I believe that he meant to tell us that we needn't worry about how we would acquire food — God will provide. Jesus went on to say that God provides for the birds and the lilies of the field, why should we concern ourselves that He won't provide for us.

God does provide life-giving foods for us. It is man who deems it wise to turn them into multicolored lumps of toxic waste.

I don't know if anyone can really describe the experience in the magic garden. It has to be lived. The gardens are everything and more than I dreamed they would be. I pray that every person on the planet will have a chance to eat and play in a magic garden.

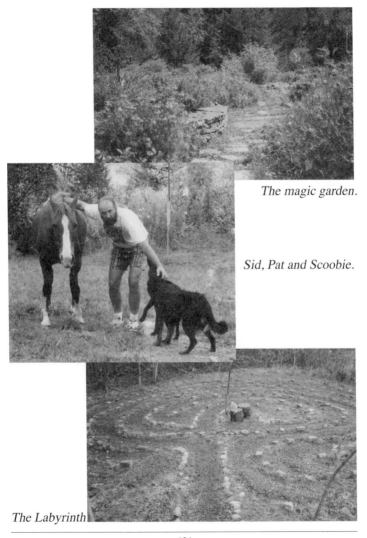

The magic garden.

Sid, Pat and Scoobie.

The Labyrinth

FOOD FOR THOUGHT...

What I wanted to share most of all through this book is the message that suPRANAtural™ foods changed the way my body and mind work and opened me up spiritually. We really are what we eat!

JUST FOR FUN...

A dietician was once addressing a large audience in Chicago:

"The material we put in our stomachs is enough to have killed most of us sitting here, years ago. Red meat is awful. Soft drinks erode your stomach lining. Chinese food is loaded with MSG. Vegetables can be disastrous and none of us realizes the long-term harm caused by the germs in our drinking water. But there is one thing that is the most dangerous of all and we all have, or will, eat it. Can anyone tell me what food it is that causes the most grief and suffering for years after eating it?"

A 75-year-old man in the front row stood up and said, "Wedding cake!"

THE SECOND COMING OF LOWELL

When I was still living with Fred, I got a call from Lowell one afternoon. By this time he was nineteen. I had received a bazillion calls from Lowell since leaving Colorado five years earlier, but this call was different. We talked about Victoria Falls in Zimbabwe for a while and then made some small talk about the weather. Actually, all conversations with Lowell were small talk, but this day he dropped something very, very big.

He said, "You know, Denise, I think I can beat this autism thing. The doctors keep saying that it isn't curable, but I don't believe that." I acknowledged that, without a doubt, autism was curable and that if he thought he could beat it, he could. That conversation lasted about five minutes and then he descended right back into small talk as if this bombshell had never been dropped. I cried for three days.

Almost exactly a year later, after I'd moved onto the farm with Pat and Patrick, I got a call from Lowell's mother. He had received some money from his grandmother, she told me, and would like to come out and visit. We arranged for him to fly out for a few days in December. He was so excited about the trip that he called constantly in the weeks prior to his arrival.

He was living on an organic farm in Fort Collins, Colorado, with a wonderful caretaker named Floyd who loved him dearly. Lowell apparently enjoyed the farm and was a good worker. Floyd's farm wasn't anything like Pat's, but he did have some chemical-free produce growing.

The problem was that Floyd would frequently drive Lowell to Dairy Queen and Denny's and other junk food havens. I understood. I had done the "babysit him with food" thing many times myself. The "babysit him with videos" strategy didn't work well with Lowell. He would talk all the way through the movie. It was hard to keep coming up with ways to hang with Lowell without going crazy. I love you, Lowell. It's the autism that's hard to handle.

Normally I got very anxious when Lowell was coming out to visit, but this time he would only be staying for two and a half days. That would be perfect, enough time for a fun visit but not enough time to cost me valuable brain cells.

I felt like a mother waiting for her son to return from his first semester of college as Pat and I headed for the airport. Pat had heard all the Lowell stories by now and was still unprepared for the depth of the being he was about to meet.

Lowell's mother had had to dump him at the airport early and take off because a huge blizzard was moving in and she had a sixty-mile drive home. Due to the weather conditions, the airline had decided to put Lowell on an earlier flight than the one he was booked on. They had tried to contact us, but we had gone out for dinner before leaving for the airport, so we had no idea that he had already arrived.

As we entered the terminal I heard them paging me. Lowell had been sitting in the back room of the ticket counter for hours. He came bounding out when he heard my voice. The folks at the counter seemed happier to see me than Lowell did. My guess was that they were all now quite versed on the geography of Zimbabwe.

He looked so grown up and mature. Although his stature hadn't changed much, he looked older and more "normal." Lowell was blossoming into a very handsome young man who still had a boyish essence. He and Pat seemed to hit it off right away.

Lowell and I swapped stories about "the good old days" all the way home. He was incredible with dates. He'd say something like, "Remember that day that we went to the civic center and blah blah blah?"

I'd say, "Gee, Lowell, my memory isn't quite as sharp as yours, why don't you remind me."

"It was November 4th, 1997, and we..." Mind you, this wasn't some monumental day in his life he was reminiscing about. It was just a typical day when we had hung out together. He had an exact date for just about every memory he had. I'm lucky if I can remember the time of an event within a five years.

Lowell was having some physical problems as a result of seventeen years of prescription drugs. According to his sister, the doctors had started him on Ritalin when he was three years old, and he had been on a combination of drugs ever since. When he visited us he was taking Tegretol and Zoloft and had been on them for years. Terrible facial tics and acne plagued him and his digestive tract was shot.

I looked up Tegretol in the 1993 Physician's Desk reference. It is such a dangerous drug that the PDR recommended that a person on this drug should be evaluated monthly and should not be on it for over a year. One of the possible side effects listed was fatal heart disease!

Tegretol is an antiseizure drug. Lowell did not have a problem with seizures. He should never have been on this life-threatening medication, yet he had been given this drug for years with little or no medical supervision.

It was not his family doing this. It was the system. When the government contributes money to support a special-needs person, they dictate that person's life.

We called Lowell's mother and told her that we felt the drugs were literally killing Lowell. We recommended that she let us detox him and get him on some herbs and a whole foods diet. She excitedly agreed. Deb Stucklen, Lowell's mother, had dedicated most of her adult life to trying to find a way to help Lowell. She hated the drugs, but the doctors convinced her that she wouldn't be able to handle Lowell without them.

By the time Lowell flew home, just two and a half days later, he was a totally different guy. His facial tics were almost gone, his skin was clearer and he was thinking and speaking like a functioning adult much of the time. He still had a long ways to go, of course. He still had loops of talking about the same old stuff, but he could control it more easily.

I could say, "Gee, Lowell, I'm kind of tired of Zimbabwe. Could we talk about something else?"

He'd say, "Sure, Denise," and search his memory banks for another topic. It required my helping his brain shift gears, but at least he could do it.

The day before he left, Lowell talked with his mother on the phone. When I got on the phone with her she was in tears. "It's a miracle," she cried.

We sent Lowell home with a set of diet recommendations, some nutritional supplements, and some "vibrational" herbs. I felt these particular herbs had changed my life significantly and they were definitely a factor for Lowell. Joseph Montagna, the herbalist who had developed these vibrational herbs, had combined herbs and minute amounts of crystals to address very specific issues or dysfunctions. There are 360 of them, designed by categories of physical ailments or emotional or spiritual challenges. (www.alternativescentral.com)

We are all just vibrations, moving molecules. Each thought and each physical manifestation has its own vibrational frequency. These herbs help us shift our vibrations to healthy ones — good vibes instead of bad vibes, you might say.

Hardly coincidentally, Lowell was about to become homeless. Floyd was selling his farm and they hadn't been able to find a new group home for Lowell. And Pat and I were trying to find a way to make a living with our healing work.

It appeared that God was listening intently to all of us. Lowell's grandmother put up $10,000 for him to stay with us. He would be returning to us in approximately a month. The problem was there were already three of us living in a one-and-a-half bedroom house. We would have to add some housing for Lowell.

If we had had more time, things could have turned out differently. We had originally planned to build a straw-bale house for Lowell. We thought that we could do it for about $3000 and then have enough money left over to support Lowell and ourselves for about six months. Unfortunately, Pat didn't own this farm; he leased it from Sydney Willett, who was a Baptist missionary in Taiwan. Sydney was worried about the effect on her property taxes and nixed the straw-bale house idea.

By the time Lowell arrived we still hadn't come up with housing for him. He would have to camp on the couch for a few weeks. We looked at buying him a Yurt. A Yurt is a very sophisticated tent-like structure. They are round, have a high ceiling with a clear dome on the top, supported by wooden lattice work, with windows and a wooden door. The insulation was designed by NASA to radiate your body heat back at you, and they sit on a wooden platform supported by cement footings. Yurts are movable, so they don't impact the property taxes as long as you don't plumb them.

In the weeks prior to Lowell's second coming, I was a wreck. I loved Lowell and I wanted this opportunity to help him get his life back. I also wanted this chance to establish our healing business. But the prospect of spending twenty-four seven with Lowell was overwhelming. Lowell is an intense being and his concentrated focus was always on me.

Pat kept saying, "Oh, stop worrying about it. I can handle him."

In my frustration I would bark back, "You're in denial. Two days with him was nothing. You have no idea what we're in for." Pat saw me as a hysterical woman. He had run day cares, raised his own son and taught Sunday school, but none of that stacked up to caring for Lowell full-time. By the time Lowell returned in mid-January (I'm sure Lowell could tell us the exact date), I was a mess and quite angry with Pat.

Nonetheless, we were very excited about Lowell's arrival. What an opportunity to show the world that the doctors are dead wrong when they tell somebody that their challenge is permanent. All things are possible with faith. Lowell had faith that he could conquer his autism and he had manifested two people who shared that faith and who knew how to help him beat his dis-ease.

I was beginning to find out that that's how God works. If you know what you want, all you have to do is ask for it, have faith that you will get it, and let the Universe handle the details. The Bible says, "Ask and you shall receive." It is my belief that every thought we have, every phrase we utter, and each action we do is a prayer. If I run around whining, "I'll never get that job," I probably won't, because that is the command I gave the Universe. Therefore, we must be religious about putting out positive thoughts and deeds (and of course, putting in whole foods and pure water).

We had formulated a plan to get Lowell to the finest alternative health professionals we knew. Pat was the expert on food, and I knew how to help people reclaim their personal power and deal with their rage. We wanted Lowell to have the best healers in every other category too.

Lowell's family had not been able to maintain the strict diet guidelines we had given them, so he had been back on the toxic foods and the dangerous drugs in the month he was home. He had slid back a ways physically and a little bit emotionally, but we were very pleased to find that he had held onto a lot of his mental clarity.

The first thing we did was to take him to Badeish Lange for a reading. She told us two profound things about Lowell that turned out to be significant. She said that he had sounds trapped inside him and that the didgeridoo would benefit him a lot. She also told us that he was going to be a writer someday and that he should start a journal and write every day.

The writer part really came out of the blue because, although Lowell can converse like an adult on some topics, his writing skills were about first grade level. But, sure enough, after we bought him a journal, he dove into the writing.

When we did didgeridoo treatments on Lowell he would start singing his feelings as we played. He loved the didgeridoo and requested treatments all day every day. It also seemed to bring him some relief for the physical pain he was experiencing in his feet and helped him sleep.

We took him to Dorothy (my recent ex-roommate, who had a masters in education) to run some diagnostics on him to see exactly what his educational levels were. She also did some other-dimensional work on Lowell, removing some earth-bound spirits from his aura. We put

Lowell to work on his language and penmanship skills and bought him some books and educational toys.

Next stop was Joseph Montagna's store, Atlantis Rising, to get Lowell and Pat and me some vibrational herbs. We picked out a number of remedies to help Lowell with his physical and emotional challenges, and Pat and I each picked out herbs for our own personal needs. As caregivers we have to take care of our own issues and continue on in our growth in order to help those in our care. Did we ever! One cannot hang with Lowell without being emotionally and spiritually stretched. Thanks, Lowell!

Finally, we shopped for organic foods and nutritional supplements. Pat laid out a diet, herb and supplement schedule for Lowell and I got him started on some rage work. We scheduled didgeridoo sessions each day, massaged Lowell's hands and feet, and spent endless hours talking and walking and listening with Lowell.

So many extraordinary things happened in the three and a half months that followed that I am overwhelmed with the task of telling you about it and getting this book to press in under a thousand pages. In a nutshell, it was a wild spiritual and emotional ride for all of us!

Pat found out before long that he had underestimated what all day, every day with Lowell would entail, especially for me. Each morning started with Lowell sitting patiently on the couch, staring at the bedroom door, waiting for me to emerge.

Lowell was every bit as intense as Shadow was when stalking a field mouse, and I was his prey. He wanted my full attention every waking moment of the day, and he peered into the depths of my soul. No superficial relationship would do; he expected every ounce of my consciousness. God forbid I had to go to the bathroom after rising. Lowell would follow me in. I would have to ask him to wait in the living room for a moment.

A day with Lowell was like spending a week with a room full of six-year-olds, only there was no quiet time and they asked one question after another and they didn't go home at the end of the day. The questions and the intense focus went on until bedtime (which was quite early, as you can imagine).

One of the greatest things that Joseph's herbs did for Lowell was to help him control some of his obsessive habits. We got him a vibrational remedy specifically for excessive talking. (Actually, we bought it for the preservation of our own sanity, but we administered it to Lowell.) With this herb, he could sit quietly for hours if you got him settled. Previously, he couldn't stop talking no matter how much you begged. It was simply out of his control.

His bowels started working better and his skin improved daily. He also started to put on a little weight. Interestingly, every person we have detoxed either dropped their excess weight or put on some needed pounds — all on the same diet. Whole foods seem to balance the body so that it can right itself.

The rage therapy also had a deep effect on Lowell, but it took a while before he got to his reservoir of stored anger. Rage therapy, the way I teach it, is controlled violence with the express purpose of dissipating old, stored emotions.

For Lowell we took all the glassware that we were going to recycle and labeled each bottle with the name of a person, event, or in Lowell's case, a place that made him angry. Lowell made the labels and glued them on the bottles himself. Then we took the batch to the recycling center and hurled the bottles into the appropriate bins while shouting the name of the person, event or place that had caused him pain or anger in the past.

The first few times we did this he giggled and had fun with it, but one day when Pat took him to the center he really got in touch with some old feelings. When Pat walked away for a moment to go get more ammunition out of the car, Lowell cut loose. He was throwing the bottles with such intensity and furry that some of the glass was landing in the parking lot and endangering people. Pat reported that he looked like a crazed animal and that it was quite a chore to pull him out of it. Later that day, Lowell was more relaxed and at peace than we had ever seen him.

When we ran out of bottles, we would take him outside, put safety glasses on him, and let him pummel bricks with a hammer. While tapping into his "stuff" on the bricks one day, he became manic with rage and began beating a tree with his hammer. Lowell loves nature, and when he was reminded of that fact he was able to pull out of it. But he had successfully shown us how big his reservoir was.

After that, when he was feeling frustrated or stuck I would recommend some rage therapy. "Yeah, Denise," he would say, "I think I better hit a few bricks. I think I'm feeling kinda mad."

It was the first time in Lowell's life that he was allowed to feel angry. Every other time he had tried to express his rage and frustration he had been punished or sedated. Autism is a frustrating dysfunction; it would certainly drive me to violence.

Shortly after arriving, Lowell began to tell us about some incidents of physical and sexual abuse in his past. I was shocked and surprised that he had never told me before, until I found out that every time he had tried to tell someone about these incidents, he had gotten slammed. They had presumed he was lying or telling stories just for attention, and he had been either dismissed or sedated. The system is not well prepared for such disclosures. I made enough calls around Colorado to substantiate Lowell's claims.

The validation that Lowell received from us changed him. Nobody wants to believe that rapes and assaults happen, but denying them just revictimizes the survivor. Lowell blossomed very quickly after sharing that information and getting supported.

I tried to walk him into some beliefs about his autism one day, to give him some comfort as to why he had lost twenty years of his life to this monster. I don't remember what I said to him, but this is verbatim what he said to me: "That's not it, Denise. I chose autism before I came here as a means to cope with what I knew was going to happen, and I don't need it anymore."

I was blown away. In a matter of weeks we had gone from ten years of discussion about water slides and Zimbabwe to conversations about reincarnation and coping mechanisms. He started spouting all kinds of spiritual and philosophical ideas.

We wanted to make sure that this miracle got documented, so we let him loose on our phone, allowing him to talk to every caretaker, psychiatrist, family member and friend who had ever known him around the country. They were all as dumbstruck as I was.

Lowell loved the labyrinth. Sometimes he would go out there and walk for hours. He felt that special something out there that Pat, Betty, the animals and I had all discovered.

Lowell's twenty-first birthday was coming up. That date I definitely remember, February 13th. Lowell had a special request for his birthday. He wanted the three of us to walk the labyrinth naked. He felt that people were too hung up about their bodies, and he wanted an affirmation that bodies are beautiful gifts from God that we shouldn't be ashamed of. Cool theory, but not so easy in practice.

Lowell was fine with it, but Pat and I were a mess. Nonetheless we thought it would be a good experience. It was one of the many opportunities to stretch that Lowell had brought into our lives. Stretch we did. I was to find out that I am not at all comfortable in my body yet. I thought I had tamed that demon — apparently not.

I was concerned that this exercise would fuel Lowell's obsession with me, but it seemed to have the opposite effect. It strengthened our friendship and transmuted his infatuation with me into something deeper and less suffocating.

Perhaps you've noticed that this chapter isn't full of cute, endearing stories like the last chapter about Lowell. It was a really hard time for us. We needed more help and more money to take care of Lowell. Even with two of us trading him off, we were worn out by the end of the day. The Yurt ended up costing us $7000, and we spent a lot of money right off the bat to get Lowell started in the right direction.

Grandma had said that she had a trust fund for Lowell, and should we need more money just ask. We presumed that when she saw how fast he was progressing there would be no problems. But she couldn't understand how we had spent all that money in two months. Grandma cut us off. The last month that Lowell stayed with us we were writing hot checks for groceries and borrowing from Peter to pay Paul. We were all worn down to the nub by the time we decided that Lowell would have to return to Colorado.

I am sick to have to tell you that the system put him right back on drugs and toxic food. Just about any government agency that deals with special-needs people has psychiatrists on board. Their philosophy seems to be to keep people heavily sedated so that they don't get overwhelmed by their emotions and so that the caregivers can stand to be around them. They also feed them toxic treats all day to keep them happy.

The good news is that Lowell has hung on to most of his mental clarity and knows how he would like to eat and drink when he gets the chance to make his own choices. We continue to pray for the funds to invite Lowell back and work with him again in grand style. We love you, Lowell!

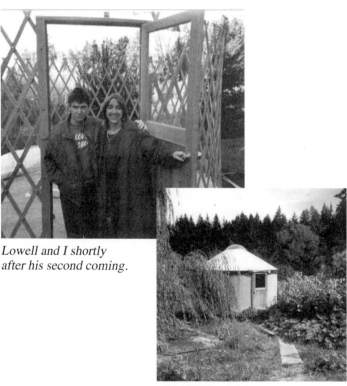

Lowell and I shortly after his second coming.

The finished Yurt by the Magic Garden.

FOOD FOR THOUGHT...

Those three and a half months with Lowell were the most emotionally demanding of my life to date. But Lowell showed us what was possible and forced us to peer into our own souls.

The fact that the food and herbs had such an enormous effect on Lowell didn't surprise me. Like all autistic people, he is a very sensitive person. Chemicals, sugar, steroids, dyes and flavorings are heavy poisons to him.

What I want to know is this: What was the driving event that spurred Lowell to call me and say, "I think I can beat this autism thing." That could be one of the crucial keys to human evolution. In other words, we can't help anyone until they find the faith and the courage to face their mountain. Against all odds, including the beliefs of a vast team of medical and psychiatric professionals, Lowell had found that special something that led him to believe he could find his way out of autism. If he could tell us what brought him to that belief, perhaps we could help millions of others make that leap of faith.

Once again, the trick is to recognize when your prayers have been answered. They don't always look the way we expect them to. Lowell was truly an answered prayer for us and we were for him, even though his presence didn't always feel like a blessing. Working for the greatest good is not always comfortable or easy, but it is definitely worth the effort.

JUST FOR FUN...

Have you heard about the old geezer who wouldn't vacate his home when the floods came? The Sheriff sent a pickup over to get him.

"Come on Jed. The river is rising, you're gonna have to evacuate your house."

Jed replied, "God will save me. I ain't leavin'."

A few hours later the water was pouring over the front porch. The Coast Guard sent a boat over for Jed. Once again, Jed vehemently declared, "God will save me. I ain't leavin'."

By sundown Jed was standing on the roof. The Air Force sent a helicopter over for Jed. Jed shouted up at the chopper, "God will save me. I ain't leavin'."

Jed drowned. By the time he got to the pearly gates he was not a happy camper. He gave St. Peter a piece of his mind.

"I had so much faith that God would save me that I refused to leave my home in a flood and I drowned. Why didn't God help me?"

St. Peter replied, "We sent you a pickup, a boat and a chopper. What more did you want?"

An old classic

It Can't Be Denial...
I Never Said That

It was a slow beginning with Pat, but eventually we fell very much in love. As I mentioned earlier, Pat and I did a lot for each other. He gave me a home, a lot of love and showed me how wonderful it could be to be with a man who was warm, sensitive and emotional. Pat also kept me out of the grave. He helped me beat my addictions by cooking for me and educating me about food.

Pat would sometimes spend hours happily chopping, steaming, and preparing delicious, life-affirming meals. He would rub my back and feet and lay his healing hands on me, and he was always eager to jump up and get anything I asked for. He put his son, Patrick, first (as it should be) and he almost always put my needs before his own (not good).

Everybody loved Pat, even when they didn't like hearing his sermons. I, however, had a different effect on people, sometimes evoking genuine rage, perhaps because I still had plenty inside me.

In our relationship, Pat was always the first to apologize and try to bring the conversation back to love. He could be so loving at times that he'd overwhelm me and I would react negatively. I had never met someone so deeply loving before and I didn't trust that his feelings were real.

To me his love; didn't feel like a sexual love or a romantic love; I had encountered those before. Pat's love poured out from him to all beings, like the love of a minister for his congregation.

I would talk to Pat about the fact that his outpouring of love was too much for me. His face would soften with that reverent smile of his and he'd say, "I know." But he kept exposing me to it in the hope that someday he would penetrate my armor and reach me. Pat was a wonderful, gentle, person, most of the time.

Unfortunately, this warm, fuzzy, lovable guy had a dark side, which brought out a very dark side of me. He might say something to me as innocent as "I fed Sid," and then an hour later come out with "I better go feed Sid."

I'd remind him, "But you said you already fed him."

That could be all it took to trigger an angry defense from him.

"No I didn't! I never said that!"

Sometimes he'd abandon logic, giving a long-winded soliloquy on his point of view and then jump to the other side of the argument without explanation. If I dared ask him what he meant by what he had said first, he would batter me with "I never said that."

Gone was that reverent smile and loving demeanor. And gone was my sense of mental and emotional equilibrium.

Whether it was trivial stuff or critical issues that triggered these incidents, it felt as if Pat was systematically trying to drive me insane. Sometimes I thought his behaviors were calculated, but most of the time it was obvious to me that he wasn't conscious of what he was doing at all. My gift to Pat was to help him see, and break through, this pattern of denial. It drove us both to the brink of our sanity.

If I am not listening or am uninterested, I can have a memory lapse, but in general I have an impressive memory, except for dates and time frames, and of course some of the traumatic events from childhood. I can usually tell you which direction I was facing and what you were wearing when you said it. My memories come most often in the form of pictures. I usually have a still photo to go with the verbal message.

The "I never said that" episodes happened almost daily. Every few days or so an exchange would blow up into an ugly argument. I was not going to let him convince me that I was crazy. I knew what I had heard and I wasn't about to back up on it. We would get into screaming battles. I would bark, "You're in denial," and he would shout, "No I'm not, you are!"

Sometimes I could bombard him with enough evidence that he would realize that he indeed had said "it," whatever "it" was this time. Sometimes our arguments would escalate until one of us started screaming at the top of our lungs, one of us punched or kicked a wall in frustration, or one of us took off.

I was usually the one to leave. I would cry, bitch, scream and finally in my frustration shout, "Screw you!" and take off walking. Once in a while I would take off in the truck. I spent many nights sitting in the woods or an abandoned house or the barn until I had calmed down enough to come back.

My leaving usually made Pat manic. He could be hurling cutting insults at me one minute and sobbing violently the next. His core issue in life is abandonment; mine is denial. For that reason we could be an explosive duo. On a couple of occasions our encounters became violent.

One such night I had gotten in the truck and was headed down the gravel road that led to the farm. Pat chased me, grabbed my hair through the open window and got me in a headlock. I clawed his face while I drove the truck into a tree. The truck got a dent, Pat had scratch marks on his face, and I ended up with a sore neck. It was a miracle we survived this craziness.

There were a couple of factors to this madness that bear mentioning. Anytime we backed off the processed foods it would stimulate a detox. Besides purging the physical toxins, a mountain of toxic emotions would surface too. Pat and I were in a heavy detox at this time as we had been primarily eating out of the garden. Once Lowell came we all jumped into an intense detoxification program, including a variety of herbs and supplements. Detoxing can precipitate an emotional roller coaster. It certainly did with the three of us, facing a lifetime worth of baggage, all at once, in a tight space.

The other factor was the stress level. Handling Lowell on a daily basis was always a stretch and the bills were a constant recurring nightmare. Pat and I were in overload all the time. We were both ticking bombs.

We had a couple of these battles when Lowell was with us. Lowell would always side with me. Every now and then Lowell would find the courage to tell Pat he was in denial. That didn't go over real big with Pat and caused a rift between them. On principle, I wanted Lowell out of the middle, but I have to admit it was nice to have an ally once in a while.

The week of Lowell's birthday was one of the wildest times of my life. I was embarking on a spiritual high that was to spur a quantum leap in my awakening.

Besides my other 682 dysfunctions, I also still struggled with my sleep disorder. I sometimes went days without dozing off at all. I now understand that those sleep deprivation stretches were caused by dehydration. Our adrenal glands are our 911 agency; they switch into emergency status when something is out of balance in the body.

My adrenal glands would go into survival mode when I got dehydrated. If I had been in the wilderness, this would have kept me awake for an extended period of time so that I could find water. In real life, it just kept me awake. So I worked more, which would use up more water, consequently stimulating my adrenal glands. Sleep deprivation was a vicious cycle for me, and a drug. Once I got going on one of these sleepless rolls, I didn't want to stop. It felt very much like a speed trip.

By the time we took that naked hike through the labyrinth for Lowell's birthday, I was on day five of what would become a six-day sleep deprivation binge. I had slept maybe three hours in the previous five days. It was also one of those stretches when I was hearing God's voice loud and clear. Every single thing I saw was a symbol or had a purpose, and I was desperately trying to keep up with the rush of information.

The night before Lowell's birthday Pat and I had gotten into one of those "I never said that" arguments. We were in the vicious name-calling stage in our bedroom when Pat tackled me. We were rolling around on the floor. He wasn't trying to hurt me, just control me, which was a very bad idea. I threatened to hurt him real bad, shoved him off me, and took off towards the front door.

Pat followed me to the front stoop, saying something like "Just go ahead and kill me, that's what you want anyway."

This scenario was something I had feared for many years. I had some very deadly skills, and I also knew that I still had my share of stored rage. I had always wondered: If somebody pushed me too far, would I be able to control my rage or would I accidentally kill them and end up in prison for the rest of my life? I was about to find out.

Pat came lunging at me again. I remember that second of my life better than anything in my memory banks. It all seemed to happen in slow motion. I thought,

"Well, I can kick him up under his jaw, snap his neck and kill him. I can throw a hook kick at his face and break his jaw or I can kick him in the chest and just knock him down."

I opted to just knock him down. If he got back up and came at me again, I would start from scratch and re-evaluate my choices. This whole process seemed to take forever, one frozen frame at a time. I picked up my leg, tucked it, aimed at his chest, and delivered a blow. Pat fell to the ground. He decided to back off.

Seeing that I could stay controlled under that much pressure was a great gift for me. I was now confident that I could control my skills and my rage. Pat claims that that moment was a significant turning point in his life as well. He had physically assaulted women before, but he was in denial about it. He could now see how wrong it is to take advantage of someone because you are bigger or stronger. He could finally admit that he had done it, and he says that he is grateful to have found a woman who could "kick his ass" so he could "get it," so to speak.

There is a difference between lying and denying something. A lie is when you purposefully tell an untruth. You know what the truth is, but you are choosing not to go with it. Denial is when you are hiding the truth from yourself. The information is in your brain, but you can't get to it. That is why intervention is so important when dealing with addicts. They often can't face their behaviors or change them (so they think), so they go into denial about what they are doing in order to deal with the shame.

Leaving a friend in a self-destructive pattern because it is uncomfortable to confront them on their denial is not true friendship. Using my definition, a true friend is one who will risk the friendship to save the friend.

Helping Pat see what he was doing was my initial motive, but eventually it turned into all-out psychological warfare. I thought he was trying to drive me insane and he thought that I was trying to make him feel stupid. Our "I never said that" exchanges took on a life of their own that consumed us. My birthday is January 27th and Lowell's is February 13th. We usually picked a date in the middle to celebrate. This year we had decided to have our joint party on his birthday. It would also be a party for my attorney friend Joel, whose birthday is January 28th. Pat had tried to round up about twenty people and Joel and I had put the word out too. We didn't give these people much notice, and Pat and I weren't that popular anyway as we were always preaching about food.

I arranged displays all over the house about healthful eating habits, children's safety, and denial. I thought it would be a great opportunity to educate our friends and family. If they wanted to look at the materials they could. If they didn't want to they could frolic on the farm or enjoy the campfire and the labyrinth. Pat and I and Joel and Lowell were the only people who showed up for the party.

I had enjoyed my romp on Sid's back that day and survived our stroll through the labyrinth, so it wasn't a total bust, but I was angry and disappointed.

I had also received a package from Michael Eisner's office at Disney that day. It wasn't great news, but since I was celebrating my birthday and I felt so plugged into God, I considered it an affirmation that the deal would eventually go through; I thought it would just require patience and finesse.

We decided to take Lowell up to The Happy Fortune restaurant for dinner and a beer. We figured one beer wouldn't kill Lowell and he wanted that rite of passage that most of us crave on our 21st Birthday. But while we were there Pat told the owner, Michael, a friend and a business associate of mine, that I was "losing it." That enraged me. I thought Pat was losing his mind, since he often couldn't remember from moment to moment what he had just said.

I couldn't face another argument with Pat, so I took off walking from the restaurant. I walked to the house of a close friend we had invited to the party. When she opened the door, I demanded an explanation as to why she hadn't come to my party after she had called and said she was on her way.

She gave me a line of bull and tried to invite me in. I refused. "I want an explanation and a ride home," I demanded. "I'll be walking northeast towards Scholls-Ferry road." She apparently called the police and told them that I was suicidal. Admittedly, I was very tired. But I was stone-cold sober, drug-free, and angry, not suicidal.

I started walking down the median of the road. I was hoping a cop would see me and drive me home. I was physically and mentally exhausted.

Within a few minutes a cop passed me going the other direction. I flagged him down. When he stopped I calmly stated, "I need some help." He told me not to move. I have had a lot of experience with the police because of my crisis intervention work. I knew exactly what to do to gain his support.

I stopped dead in my tracks and waited for him to pull a U-turn. When he approached me I answered all his questions coherently and told him that I was very tired and just needed a ride the last mile to my farm.

He said, "That's funny, I just got an APB (all points bulletin) on you saying that you are suicidal."

I laughed. I convinced him that I wasn't suicidal, just pissed off at my friend. He drove me home. No one was home when we arrived. He was so convinced that I was legit that he refused to come in and let me prove it to him.

He looked me square in the eyes and said, "I know who you are." I asked him if I could have his name so that I could include this incident in my book on denial. His name was Officer John Featherstone. Thanks, John! Eventually Pat and Lowell came back. After we put Lowell to bed Pat and I got into it again. I should have recognized that Pat was going down from sleep deprivation. Although he had had much more sleep than I at this point, his mind was breaking down. I was quite experienced with these five-day sleepless rolls, but Pat couldn't handle one night without rest.

This next battle dragged us all over town in the middle of the night, created another police action which I managed to dissipate, and culminated with Pat breaking down into a sobbing pile in the parking lot of Safeway at 4:00 am. Pat thought I was losing my mind. I thought he was losing his. And I'm sure we both seemed quite nuts to all who encountered us that week. That is how dramatic the change in our consciousness had been. The sudden, extreme detox had brought up a mountain of emotions that overwhelmed us. Coming off toxic foods can be as severe emotionally as going cold turkey from heroin.

In spite of all the ugliness between us, Pat had bought me a bouquet of Valentine flowers while at Safeway, just moments before his breakdown. The demons in him couldn't keep his loving nature in check for very long.

Although Pat outweighed me by about sixty-five pounds at the time, I managed to get him in the truck, get him home and tuck him into bed. I then went about my latest project, expanding the displays all over the house. I wanted to take pictures of all this material for an article I intended to write about abuse and denial.

Despite the high emotions and physical strain on my mind and my body, I could be quite functional after two, three, even four days of no sleep. I could find a second, third or fourth wind and tackle yet another project. I also received some of my greatest inspirations while on these sleepless highs. It was definitely another drug for me.

While I was working on my latest project that night, something weird was going on with the TV. It would only work intermittently. (No, it wasn't Bob the turtle!) During one of the brief periods that it came on I heard a news story that said President Clinton would be landing in Portland in a few hours to survey the flood damages.

I decided on the spur of the moment that I wanted to try to get the President's attention and create a news story about child abuse. My thinking was, if I could just generate a story of any kind, perhaps Mr. Clinton would catch me on the news and be sympathetic to my cause.

It was around 7 a.m. now, Valentine's Day morning. It might help you to understand my mindset, to know that I had been trying persistently for fifteen years by then to distribute information about abuse prevention. I had found that the press and the police only reacted to tragedy and they rarely offered information on how to prevent crimes.

I was $50,000 in debt from trying to do something about the problem of child abuse, disillusioned, angry and too proud to give up.

My father had told me that in his role as a strike negotiator, the press had been his worst enemy. Things always got stirred up when the media showed up. To hear David tell it, the press weren't interested in a sedate little strike; they wanted a story. I decided that I was willing to sacrifice my freedom for an afternoon to give them a story if it would give me a forum to talk about prevention.

Our phone lines were down from the storm that had caused all the flooding, so I had to walk to the neighbor's house to use the phone. I called my friend Ambassador Kabir. He said that he didn't have the connections to get me on the Secret Service list to see the

President. He loved me, but was worried about my state of mind. I told him to try anyway and hung up.

I thought about calling Bob Duggan, who owns Executive Security International, thinking his people might be handling some of the security for the President, but didn't have his number on me. I finally decided just to head for the airport and wing it. I figured at the very least the press would be there and I could make something happen through them. I had a rolling flight bag full of marketing materials, my correspondence with Disney, and the materials that Humayan had delivered to Hillary Clinton for me.

I was sporting my "It's A Jungle Out There" T-shirt and my "Save the Children" tie. I was also carrying my Valentine flowers.

Pat and Lowell and I headed for the airport. Pat still thought I was delirious, but he was doing everything I asked him to do. Actually, he says now that part of him loved what I was doing and part of him thought I had "gone round the bend." He didn't have enough emotional reserves to fight anymore. Lowell was just thrilled to be out for the ride.

There was no sign of President Clinton at the airport. We tried a private airport, but no deal. I decided to go forward with my plan of creating a news story, hoping President Clinton might catch me on the local news and respond. At the very least I was hoping to get the attention of Portland's Chief of Police, Dr. Charles Moose.

We headed to Perigon Communications in Beaverton, home of Channel 32. The manager of the station, Victor Ives, was slated to do the voice-overs on the SAVVY! Safety Series audiotapes which were to be recorded in their studios. I had never met Victor in person, but we had developed a lot of respect for one another through our mutual friend, Larry Anderson.

I began laying out my marketing materials all over the sidewalk in front of their main entrance. I told the receptionist to get a camera and the police. I softly informed her that I was prepared to go to jail to generate a story on child abuse prevention.

A man came out and introduced himself as Victor Ives. I excitedly hailed, "Victor!" and jumped in his arms. He was a bit surprised, but loved what I was doing. Without much ado, he headed inside to find a camera and call the police. Channel 32 had recently gone off the air so they didn't have any television cameras or crews. Unbeknownst to me, Victor got on the phone with his daughter at KOIN (another local station) and tried to get a film crew. They were all out chasing the President, but Victor somehow coughed up a camcorder and a crew and got the police on the way.

Meanwhile, Lowell and I were standing in the middle of traffic on Western Avenue. There was plenty of room for the traffic to pass us safely. I was doing this to make sure that Victor took me seriously and to generate a story worth filming. In some ways it was all a big game to Lowell, but deep inside it seemed he was glad to be part of the mission, as a person who himself had been abused.

As soon as I saw the camera, I returned to the building and did everything I was asked to do from there on out. I gave an eloquent speech about the issues I was trying to address and the denial that was perpetuating this problem. Victor and his crew were duly impressed. The cops seemed annoyed but were cooperative. They filmed me going off in handcuffs while Pat and Lowell packed up my marketing stuff and headed to the jail. Somehow the two most important documents didn't get packed. Victor ended up with them.

On the way to the police station, Officer Jaques ranted about what a maniac I was.

I smiled and spoke calmly, "Why don't you just look at the evidence before you decide who I am?"

He continued to rant, calling me an idiot, a lunatic, you name it. I bring out the best in people, wouldn't you say?

Officer Jaques put me in a holding cell, verbally assaulting me the whole time. I was calm and cooperative and kept insisting that I was a professional on a mission.

Sergeant Gary Dodson came in. Mike Jaques took him out in the hall. I could hear their conversation. Mike tried to convince his boss that I was a lunatic. Sergeant Dodson came back into the room and started the same verbal assault. I kept trying to tell him my story, but after a few minutes I was worn out. I looked Sergeant Dodson square in the eyes and declared, "Fuck You!" Amazingly, something in him shifted on the spot.

He relented. "Okay, I give. You are who you say you are. I think what you're doing is great. What can I do to help you?"

I told him I had briefly met the Chief of Police a few months back. "He has seen some SAVVY! materials and I think he cares about this cause. I am trying to get his attention, as well as generate a news story."

"I'm not denying what you're saying, Denise," the sergeant said. "I'm telling you that I'm not powerful enough to help you. If you want to get to Dr. Moose, you need to go do this in Portland."

"Great, get me out of here," I beamed.

My new friend Officer Jaques expedited the procedure. I walked in thirty minutes, with a ticket for disorderly conduct. I gave Gary Dodson my SAVVY! sunglasses as a souvenir. As he escorted me out, Pat spotted him. It turned out they were old high school chums.

On to Portland to stage my next arrest. I picked the KOIN building. Unfortunately, I didn't remember that a man had held a bunch of people hostage at gunpoint in this very same lobby. Nor did I know that Victor had called KOIN TV.

I had a relationship with this station as well. One of the marketing firms that I was working with was owned by KOIN. The video for the SAVVY! Safety Series was slated to be filmed at the KOIN studios. Previously I had been taken on a tour of the facility and treated like a queen.

As in Beaverton, I laid out my materials all over the floor of the KOIN lobby. I sat down with Lowell and my flowers and told the receptionist to call the police. I told her that I was trying to create a news story about child abuse. A terrified man showed up and asked me to leave. Only a glass wall separated us. I politely said "I'm not leaving; please call the police."

Enter…"The Boys." When Officer Plouchos and Officer Cummins came into the KOIN lobby, I began excitedly rattling on at ninety miles an hour about my cause. Eventually, Officer Plouchos said, "Shut up! You haven't stopped talking since we walked in."

Guilty as charged, I responded with, "I'll shut up if I get a chance to respond after you're done talking."

He agreed. The next thing out of his mouth was, "I agree that anybody who doesn't think that child abuse is a problem is an abuser." I was in heaven, thinking that I had an ally. He then continued on about the fact that this was not an appropriate way to get attention for my cause. I was quietly nodding my head in agreement, waiting my turn to prove to him that I had tried every appropriate means in the Universe to get attention for my mission. When he finished I asked his permission to get down on the floor and get some materials to prove to him that I had connections to the White House and to Disney, that I wasn't just a lunatic. He agreed to let me do that.

However, unbeknownst to me, the two documents that I was looking for weren't there. I began hunting for other documents: I had plenty of stuff to show him, but Officer Plouchos started getting annoyed. By the time I found something and put it in his hands, he was doing a Mike Jaques, ranting about what a lunatic I was. He wouldn't even look at what I handed him. He just threw it to the ground. I was talking away, trying to get him to listen to me. I tried to hand him another document, which he wouldn't even take. I got pissed and flung it across the room.

He said, "That's it! We're taking her in."

Calmly, I said, "Thank you. That's all I ever asked for."

Officer Plouchos and Officer Cummins became angry and aggressive. I stayed calm. I didn't say a word. But Officer Plouchos did his best to wrench my shoulder off while Officer Cummins purposely tried to snap my left wrist in two.

I know what cops want. They want you face down on the ground so that they feel safe. I tried to slowly head for the floor, but they were hurting me so badly that I couldn't.

I was now bent over at the waist looking officer Cummins in the balls. I believed that I could take both these guys. I also believed that I would end up in prison for life, possibly missing an arm or two. I decided to stay calm. Cummins was close to snapping my wrist, and I was crying in pain.

I lifted my head up and cried, "Hey, man, you said that if I was calm you wouldn't do this."

"You're not calm!" Cummins snapped and wrenched my wrist harder.

I believe that at that moment, Officer Plouchos realized that his partner was out of control, that too many people were watching, and that this could cost him his career. (I found out later that there were many reports of excess force against Portland cops. In fact, both of these cops had other complaints against them. One women had ended up with a broken arm from one of these officers and there were reports of others with similar claims.)

All I saw, once they started hurting me, besides Cummins' crotch, was Pat's face. I was very concerned that, on seeing his girlfriend being battered, he would lose it and make matters worse. Thankfully, Pat kept his cool. He was pleading, "Hey, she's calm, you have no right to be hurting her." Lowell was right behind me. Beaverton had been fun and games to him, but this traumatized him greatly.

The Boys calmed down. I don't remember who put the cuffs on me but they clamped them down so hard that it left a deep divot in my flesh, broke the skin slightly in one spot and bruised the bone on my wrist. I also sustained a deep bruise on my left arm where Officer Cummins was squeezing the crap out of me on the way to the patrol car. I documented my injuries with photos later.

I was sitting alone in the back of the patrol car while they went back inside the KOIN building to handle the paperwork. I decided to try to attract some attention so that people would remember me when I started canvassing the area looking for witnesses for the lawsuit I would want to pursue. I looked each person who walked by the car in the eyes and said, "Remember my face. I love you."

Eventually, Officer Plouchos got in and we headed to the police station. He kept up the "You're a lunatic" diatribe the whole way. I was calm, or perhaps numb is the appropriate word. I was trying to convince him that what I was doing was no different from environmentalists chaining themselves to an endangered tree. I wasn't just recklessly breaking the law; I had an intention and an agenda. He didn't listen to a word I said.

We were now parked in a garage somewhere. I had no idea where I was. Greg (I had asked him his first name in an effort to create a more personal connection with him) was still on the verbal assault. I distinctly remember his calling me "Looney Tunes," which is one of my personal favorites. I started looking around as Greg was filling out his paperwork. My arm hurt a lot. I noticed other police cars and I got scared. Visions of Rodney King popped into my head. I was worried about other cops coming out of the woodwork and finishing me off.

I quietly inquired, "Am I safe here?"

Greg mumbled some kind of affirmative reply, but I was not convinced; I was still scared.

"Greg, if I remain calm am I safe here?"

That is the moment I think he opened his heart a tidge. He turned around, looked me in the eyes and stated, "Yes."

Greg decided to leave my flight bag in his trunk and took me inside. He was still on the verbal assault but his heart was no longer in it. I think he was having some doubts about my being the indigent lunatic that he originally had thought I was.

By this time I was not only calm, I was being pleasant to everyone and downright loving towards Greg. Pat and I believe that saying the words "I love you" to someone raises their vibrations enough to help them pull out of the muck. I figured I didn't have anything to lose. I must have laid sixty "I love you" comments on Greg in the next thirty minutes.

We ended up in a room somewhere deep inside the Portland police department. Greg was seated at a desk and I was sitting in a chair next to it.

I asked, "What can I do to make this paperwork easier for you?" I answered everything slowly and succinctly. My memory for numbers and details and my willingness to cooperate made the process go smoothly. Our conversation went something like this:

Denise: "Do you have any children?"

Greg: "Yes, four."

Denise: "I love you, Greg. You know what the truth is. Why don't you just look at the evidence before you decide who I am?"

Greg: No response.

Denise: "Come on, man, I love you. You know that what I'm trying to do here is a good thing. You know what the right thing to do is."

Greg: "I was just doing my job."

Denise: "I know you were. I love you for it. I'm just trying to do mine. Something has to be done about child abuse. Just look at the evidence I brought with me."

Denise: "Hey, that guy over there looks just like the actor that stars on The Commish. Have you ever seen that show?"

Greg: No response.

Denise: "Oh, it's great. You'd love it. It's about a loving police commissioner. Basically he puts his family before his job. It's a great show. You should check it out."

Greg: No Response.

Denise: "Gee, Greg, I'm a little worried about your children."

Greg (looking me square in the eyes with great horror): "Why?"

Denise: "Well, earlier you said that you agreed that anybody who doesn't think child abuse is a problem is an abuser." Again, he looked me square in the eyes. He energetically let me know his children were safe.

Denise: "Happy Valentine's Day. This isn't exactly how I had planned to spend mine. I've been fondled by every cop this side of the Mississippi and I haven't even made love to my boyfriend yet. Are you and your wife going to do anything special tonight?" I don't remember his response.

At one point I fell out of my chair and landed in a pile on the floor. Greg started to mumble something about my not knowing how to sit in the chair properly. I was still in very binding cuffs.

Defensively, I pointed out, "Greg, my wrists hurt so bad that I can't lean back. When I leaned forward I fell because the chair is broken."

Greg took a look and saw that the chair was indeed broken. He offered me a heartfelt apology and jumped up to get me a better chair. Greg seemed to have come around to my side.

He took my "Save the Children" tie off. I started to protest and then realized that he probably was concerned about my trying to hang myself with it. He stuffed it and my paperwork in my back pocket.

Greg led us into an elevator. He didn't tell me what was going to happen next or where we were going. While we were alone in the elevator I said, "You're going to think this is ridiculous, but after all I've been through today, the one thing that's really bothering me is that my bra strap is hanging half way down my arm. I don't suppose you would consider putting it back on my shoulder?"

Amazingly, he started to fumble under my sleeve to retrieve the elusive strap. Just then the elevator door began to open. I cried frantically, "Don't do it!" He immediately dropped his hands to his side. I didn't want to do anything to compromise him with his peers. He was now treating me with respect, and I needed him.

We seemed to be in another garage. We were walking towards the sheriff's department when I realized that I was going to be separated from Greg soon. I gave it one more try.

"Greg, it's not too late to do the right thing. I am going to start a lawsuit and I do know Roscoe Nelson. (Roscoe was a friend of Pat's and a very powerful criminal defense lawyer in Portland. He has a reputation for winning against the cops.) Your partner is going down and you know it. If you'll stand behind me, I promise I won't point the finger at you."

He stopped, looked at me and reluctantly declared, "Okay, if you promise not to name me, I'll stand behind you."

I beamed, "Deal!"

Amazingly, now in plain view of at least five deputy sheriffs, he reached under my sleeve and put my bra strap back on my shoulder. I thanked him.

Without saying another word Greg Plouchos put me in a cement room that had nothing but another door on the other side and slammed the door. I remember thinking, "Gee, that sucked." But I knew that he was overwhelmed by the position he had just been forced into.

I have a warm spot in my heart for Greg. I probably wouldn't have made it through my next ordeal if he hadn't shown me some warmth and respect.

A young deputy sheriff with a flattop haircut peeked in the window of the door. I felt like an animal in a cage. I smiled at him. I was starting from scratch again. He led me into a room full of deputy sheriffs and parked me in the middle of the room. Soon he was busily chatting with a large, nasty-looking female deputy who glared at me from time to time.

Mr. Macho motioned for me to step towards him. I didn't move. I asked, "Am I safe here?"

He was still chatting with the female deputy and said, "No." I knew that he was answering her and not me, but I still didn't have the response I wanted. I didn't move.

Annoyed now he looked up at me and barked, "I told you to come over here."

In a very powerful voice I declared, "And I asked you if I was safe here and you said no."

He immediately changed his manner to apologetic and warm and fuzzy. A few minutes later I started throwing Roscoe's name around and got the red carpet treatment.

Eventually I ended up in a jail cell. I was very thirsty and stood over the sink and drank for a long time. (I was pregnant at the time of my arrest. I lost the pregnancy a few days later, most likely from stress and dehydration.)

There was a bar of soap, a sanitary pad, a plastic mattress on a cement bench, and a pay phone in my cell. I took a sponge bath with the sanitary pad and the soap. I was barefoot, cold and tired.

I could write a whole book about that afternoon but I can sum it up fairly briefly. I had never been in jail before, didn't know what was going to happen to me, and didn't know how I would get out. I finally realized that I had created an opportunity to test how strong my faith was.

Once I accepted that test of faith, I felt a wonderful peace wash over me. I had no fear; I was joyous. All I had in that jail cell was God. It turned out to be one of the richest experiences of my life.

I wrapped the skimpy little mattress around me and slept for some time. I don't know how long I napped, but I felt fairly refreshed when I woke up. I called the house collect from the pay phone in my cell, but Pat wasn't there. I decided to call my sister in New Jersey. Her husband, Joel, answered the phone. Apparently, Pat had called Paula and told her that I had been battered by the cops. She was flying out to be there for me and would arrive in a few hours. Joel was quite anxious. How would Paula find me? Who would pick her up at the airport? I said, "Joel, Paula is a world traveler. She can certainly find her way to the jail in a cab if Pat doesn't meet her plane. Just relax."

(Note: One of my editors kept suggesting that I change the word calm throughout this story. She couldn't believe that I could have been calm under these circumstances. First of all, I convinced three different cops in twelve hours that I was a professional on a mission — I couldn't have been too hysterical. Secondly, I had planned to go to jail that day, so I had consciously worked hard on staying calm, cool and collected, in order to win the support of the police. Thirdly, I am an adrenaline junkie. Remember? I love crisis. After years of creating crises and doing crisis intervention work for others, I consider myself an expert at staying calm under extreme duress.)

I was still on a high from my afternoon with God in the cell. What I had realized was that no matter what any human does to your body, they can't rob you of your relationship with God. You can throw it away if you choose to, but nobody can take it from you. I'm sure Jesus, John the Baptist, Ghandi, Joan of Arc, the Apostle Paul and many others all had the same experience while sitting in prison. Ultimately, freedom lies in the heart!

I was touched that Paula would jump on a plane and fly three thousand miles to support me. But I wasn't thrilled that Pat had called her. I had a feeling that her presence was going to be a problem.

It seemed that nobody wanted me to emerge from that jail cell calm, cool and collected. I was supposed to be hysterical or else it would be proof positive that I had stepped over the edge, but I was on a delightful, spiritual high, soaking up the experience.

A few hours later I was released. Pat and Lowell were waiting in the lobby. Pat was somewhere between pissed and worried. I needed a hug, some support, or even an "Are you okay?" All I got was a cold look. He was worn out from spending the day with Lowell, which meant that he needed a hug more than I did. Lowell was thrilled to see me and became my only ally.

Paula arrived an hour or so later. She had listened to all Pat's stories and decided that I had lost my mind.

She wanted to tell me how screwed up I was and help me through it. I wasn't discounting that I still had issues, but I wanted her to acknowledge the life-altering experience I had just been through.

I tried to tell her my story, of what Pat had put me through with his denials. She didn't want to hear it. But the next day she got to observe Pat doing one of his "I never said that" routines when she knew he had. Finally I had a witness. I felt as if a huge weight had been lifted off my chest. Pat had almost convinced me I was crazy.

I had recently had a wicked fight with my mother. We had both said some really ugly things. I wanted to get it straightened out, but I was very anxious about making this call. Paula agreed to sit through it with me and give me some input when I hung up. Pat heard her make a commitment to stick around and listen to my end of the discussion, but as soon as I started talking to my mother Paula got up and walked out of the room.

Later that night, Pat and I went out and sat in the truck to talk and smoke a joint. Paula and Lowell had turned in early, and we didn't want to wake them. Pat had experienced a monumental breakthrough. He had risen above his denial and could see it as a cloud that periodically descended over his brain. I had my friend and lover back. We talked for hours. He began to experience the spiritual high that I had been on all week. He saw what I was seeing. My awakening had been spurred by the pure diet that I was on for the first time in my life.

He apologized for everything he had put me through and I did the same to him. All anger, jealousy and control had drained out of our relationship. We both felt that unconditional love that comes with finding your Godself and feeling at peace with your life.

I was leaning against the passenger door looking at Pat when I saw something walk by the truck.

"Did you see that?" I excitedly asked Pat.

"No," he replied.

What I thought I had seen was a set of clothing with nobody in it. The clothes that I had seen I recognized as my father's items that he wore when I was a kid. I saw him, it, this pile of clothes, whatever it was, walk towards the garden. My father had been dead for five years.

I got out of the truck and headed to the garden. When I got there I didn't see any clothes but I felt my father's presence. It was a warm, compassionate presence, not the scary, abusive man I had feared. We had a wonderful conversation that took place in my head. He apologized for what he had done to me but explained that his behaviors were to help me learn certain lessons this time around. I thanked him and told him that I forgave him and loved him. He wished me peace, gave me an energetic hug and drifted away. I felt whole for the first time in my life. I went back to the truck and told Pat about our conversation.

You are welcome to believe that I was hallucinating from the pot, but I had smoked pot off and on for twenty years at this point and not had any conversations with dead guys (except Pam Lacaruba's grandfather, and I wasn't stoned at that time). Pat believed me and was quite joyous for me. Pat is always teaching love and forgiveness. They are wonderful feelings when you are ready. No one should forgive before they are ready, however; you end up getting stuck in your rage. Forgiveness is a process. I was ready at that moment. By going to jail and practicing forgiveness there, I had freed my soul. Sounds crazy, doesn't it?

The following morning Paula had taken Lowell out for a walk, Pat was outside and I was alone in the house, sitting on the couch. I had water boiling on the stove. Oftentimes when I would boil water to steam my face, Pat would walk in and turn the water off without even asking me if I had a purpose for it. That would piss me off. On day six of an exhausting six-day roll, which included getting battered and going to jail, I was not in the mood for that. So, when Pat walked in the door I shouted from the living room, "Don't turn the water off, I'm going to steam my face."

"Okay," he responded, but to my utter amazement I heard him walk over and turn the stove off. The old nobs on our stove had a very audible click. He then waltzed into the living room and plopped down next to me on the couch like nothing had happened.

I looked at him and softly inquired, "Why did you turn the water off?"

He innocently remarked, "I didn't."

"Yes, you did, I heard you." He continued to contend that he hadn't turned the water off. So I suggested, "Let's go out to the kitchen and see."

The stove was off. Pat was flabbergasted. He knew that we were alone in the house. He knew that I had never left the couch, and he conceded that he remembered the water being on and my request when he came in. For the first time in his life he had caught himself in his own denial. He had a vague recollection of making up this whole alternate reality about walking to the cupboard on the other side of the kitchen when in actuality he had walked straight to the stove and turned it off. Pat says when he looked in my eyes he could tell that I wasn't messing with him, and he recognized that it was his brain that was playing the game. It changed his life.

The next day Pat was excitedly trying to tell Paula that he now saw through his denial. He was trying to tell her about the "water" incident. She didn't want to hear it. She was invested in believing that I was screwed up and didn't want to entertain any other theories. I thanked her later that day for coming to support me but recommended that she go home to her husband. We parted friends.

A month later we had a vicious encounter on the phone and through the mail. We haven't spoken since. It's been three years.

I wish my sister peace and I thank her for all she has done for me over the years. I don't know how she survived my antics anymore than how I have survived Pat's or he mine. We are all spirit guides for each other. Sometimes you have to let down your guard and let other people help you. That is the hardest work there is.

After the rendezvous with my father and the good-byes with my sister, I slept for days. I was at peace, thinking the denial thing with Pat had come to an end, or at least it would be the beginning of the end.

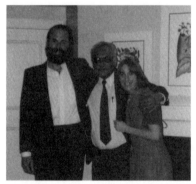

Patrick, Ambassador Kabir and myself at Humayan's hotel in Portland.

FOOD FOR THOUGHT...

Once again, what we were consuming was profoundly affecting our lives, sometimes for the good and sometimes not. I know that the consciousness that I live in when I am religious about what I consume is truly heaven. When I take care of my body, it takes care of me.

Again, attitude is the other ingredient. I try to focus on what I want, instead of what I don't have. When I eat only foods that are whole, natural, and grown in mineralized soil, it makes it easier for me to break out of negative thinking.

Forgive me for being repetitious but I can't stress this enough. We are what we drink, we are what we eat, and we are what we think and believe. In other words, when we can control what we let into our bodies through these avenues, we can write our own destiny. We truly do have the option to choose heaven on earth over hell.

JUST FOR FUN ...

A couple had identical twin girls. One was always positive and upbeat, while the other couldn't seem to find sunshine in any situation. The parents were very perplexed about this phenomenon, so they took the girls to a psychiatrist to be evaluated. The psychiatrist put the pessimistic child in a room full of toys and treats and watched as she complained about the shortcomings of each toy or snack.

The optimistic child was put in a room that was filled with nothing but manure. The psychiatrist watched in amazement as the young girl joyously hurled the manure in the air. After observing this for some time he could not contain his curiosity. He entered the room and asked the child what she was doing.

"Well," she exclaimed excitedly, "With all this manure, I figure there's got to be a pony hidden in here somewhere!"

THE SUGAR DETOX CENTER

The months following Lowell's departure were quite difficult for Pat and me. We were financially wiped out and depressed about returning Lowell to the system. We did a few landscaping jobs here and there but couldn't even come close to meeting our bills, which reminds me of one of my favorite Ghandi quips. Ghandi once told a reporter that "his people" complained that it cost them a fortune to keep him in poverty. Some could make the same comment about me. Anyway, back to the mission.

I wrote a letter to the editor of Newsweek, which they published. I was responding to a piece they had written about the Gulf War veterans. My letter read:

"Your article states that 'The evidence collected so far suggests that the Gulf War vets are no sicker than the general population.' I'd like to point out that that quote doesn't necessarily negate the Gulf Vets' claims, but merely emphasizes the fact that we as a nation are suffering from chemical poisoning. The symptoms are fatigue, headaches, stomach problems, rashes, aching joints, memory loss and tumors — any of those hit home?"

Newsweek had edited out my comments about organic farming and the need to improve the food supply, which I believe to be the major source of our being chemically poisoned. Without those comments most people wouldn't understand the point of my letter, so I set out to write a whole article, which I titled "Chemical Warfare Stateside."

One afternoon Pat and I went to the library to do some research for my article. I asked him to find William Dufty's *Sugar Blues* to look up information for me. Pat had read it twenty years earlier, but this time it really hit home. He interrupted me every few minutes to read me a passage from the book. We checked it out from the library, not knowing that it would take over our lives.

The more Pat read and the more we talked about the material, the more convinced we became that William Dufty was right. Sugar is at the base of much of the disease in the world. Sugar affects us as a highly addictive drug, which we dole out as treats for children. It is a dehydrator and an anti-nutrient and it is added to almost all refined foods. And, most of all, it creates and maintains a desperate wanting for more.

Pat recalled having researched sugar back in his cocaine days. Sugar is processed in the exact same way as cocaine, using the same ovens. Sitting side by side, powdered sugar looks identical to cocaine and is used as a cut in processed foods, just as Manitol is used to cut cocaine. For those of you who don't know what that means, many drug pushers add other, less expensive substances to their drugs to add weight, consequently netting more money. Manitol is an inexpensive powder that can be purchased in most health food stores for about four dollars a pound, compared to cocaine which costs anywhere from $22,000 to $45,000 a pound. By adding Manitol to their stash of drugs, dealers can dramatically increase their profits.

The major food processors are doing the same thing with sugar. That is why you will find sugar in spaghetti sauce, salad dressings, soy sauce, catsup, soup, yogurt, baby formula and more. It is cheaper than the foods that they add it to, so the manufacturer can stretch his products and make more money. It also facilitates getting people addicted to their particular brand.

Another concept that struck us is this: Sugar is used as a sender in many medications. Its job is to get the medication into your blood stream quickly. It must also send orange dye #30 or BHT and MSG (cancer-causing preservatives) just as quickly when one consumes a Twinkie or worse.

Pat had pretty much avoided white refined sugar for the past twenty years, save for an occasional loaf of bread or chips or something that had some sugar in it. I, obviously, was still challenged in the sucrose department. In the first week of November 1996, we decided to go totally off white refined sugar.

The day I gave up all refined sugars was the day I beat my bulimia. It was that simple, and it was that hard. I still had the urge to binge occasionally, but I could control it. The pull of the physical addiction was gone. Now when I felt the need to binge I could do it with healthier, lower-calorie foods and fight the desire to purge. Insomnia ceased to be a problem. I felt in control of my life for the first time ever, a freedom that for me is heaven!

Pat remembered reading a passage in *Sugar Blues* about schizophrenia. According to a survey that Mr. Dufty had seen, 100 percent of the schizophrenics they'd interviewed had an extremely high sugar diet. And most of them chain-smoked. Another thing Mr. Dufty talked about, which really struck us, was that cigarettes have sugar in them. The tobacco is rinsed in a 5 percent sugar solution. (That was the reported concentration twenty years ago; only the tobacco moguls would know what the concentration is now.)

We got to thinking: If smoking crack cocaine makes it way more addictive than snorting it, what would smoking sugar do? It didn't take us long to get an answer.

On November 15, 1996, we received a phone call from a friend. He was enthusiastically calling at 3 a.m. to alert us that NBC was rerunning a Dateline story on sugar and cigarettes. The experts said that when you burn sugar it turns into something called (I hope I have this right) acetylaldehyde, which in their opinion, is the most addictive substance on the planet. Combined with nicotine, the sum of the two substances is eight-fold more addicting than either standing alone. Perhaps that is why nicotine withdrawal products have a reported failure rate of 95 percent. The nicotine is only a small part of the problem.

We hunted for more information about refined sugar and found that there were plenty of books on the market expounding the dangers of our beloved habit. Everything we found agreed with the premise that white refined sugar is poison to the body, and there was frequent agreement that all processed sugars are a problem. The more we read, the more we realized that fructose, maltose, lactose and maple syrup all have the same effect on the body as white refined sugar, for the same reason — it's nearly impossible to stop at a safe dose. We're all consuming way too much of these overly sweet substances.

Pat had suspected this but was still holding onto his belief that honey and maple syrup were okay because they were not heavily processed and contain many important minerals. We were also still consuming fructose and sometimes maltose thinking they were harmless too.

A little voice in my head told me that we were wrong. The first week of December 1996 I decided to consume only fruits, grains and vegetables, which have plenty of natural sugar in them to balance our blood.

We discovered that when you take sugar from these natural foods and make a sweetener with them, it becomes too concentrated. You cannot eat enough apples to distress your pancreas before your stomach aches, but you can eat enough refined fructose to throw off your blood chemistry before you feel full. The same is true with honey. It is a highly concentrated food that was intended for bees. Chances are, they only consume a pinpoint of it at a time. A teaspoon or two a day is probably a safe dose, but once again, it's hard to do just a little.

One morning Pat and I got up and discussed our plans for the day and the future. Everything was upbeat and rosy. A few hours later I spoke with Pat again and everything had gone to hell in his mind. The only apparent thing that had changed was that he had eaten a bowl of oatmeal with a generous helping of honey on it. He got it. The honey had sent him into an emotional nosedive because of the swing of the hormones to balance his blood sugar. Pat gave up honey too.

Pat now speaks publicly about the effects of sugar, and he will tell you that giving up honey and all other forms of sugar was the most significant change he has ever made in his life. His brain started functioning more clearly, he felt better and he dropped the extra fifteen pounds he had been carrying in a matter of weeks, without even trying. Most of all, the "I never said that" incidents became much less frequent. He could retrieve data from his brain more readily.

We set up a sugar display at our farm. We had purchased 150 pounds of sugar (six twenty-five pound bags), which is the per capita consumption in this country. That average includes infants, the elderly and people like us who eat little or none. In other words, most people are consuming way more than 150 pounds, and that is only white refined sugar. It doesn't include honey, fructose, maltose, lactose and maple syrup or refined flours. Refined flours like breads, pretzels, crackers and cakes also turn into sugar in the body.

Is there any wonder that diabetes, which we spent

98 billion dollars trying to treat last year, is the number seven killer in this country or that one-half the population is overweight and over one-third of the population is obese?

We found evidence that sugar turns off the enzyme lipase in the body. Lipase is the enzyme that breaks down fat. This action, along with creating an endless craving for more, results in sugar being the major contributor to weight gain, even though it is not a high-calorie substance.

We also set up a display representing the weekly consumption of a three-year-old child on the USDA food program. The program is designed to reimburse day-care owners for some of their food costs if they will agree to feed the children what the government considers healthy meals. It was a horrifying amount of sugar. (Okay, so you hate me now for spoiling your love affair with sugar. Please finish the book anyway.)

I completed my article and faxed it to media agencies all over the country, including our local news stations. We had named our business "The Family Tree Sugar Detox Center." Pat had always called his stone and concrete business "The Family Tree." I proposed sticking the "Sugar Detox Center" on the end. I thought it would bring us some attention. Abuse was more like it.

Like everyone who thinks they have found the secret to life, whether that secret be Jesus or Buddha or whole foods, we set out to preach the good news. Boy howdy, are people passionate about their sugar! We got crucified on almost every front. A few enlightened beings shook their heads and said, "Oh yeah, sugar is poison," but even those folks were usually still consuming it in the refined foods they ate. They had just cut down on sweets.

Interestingly enough, the medical reporter from KOIN TV showed up to do a story on us, not knowing that I had been arrested in their lobby. Her name was Kris Eisenhower, a gorgeous little blond who weighs about 100 pounds soaking wet. She is a registered nurse and an admitted sugar junkie.

Kris filmed us, our display, and listened to the whole rap about the dangers of sugar. I handed her a file the size of War and Peace with the research we had done.

The last thing she said to me before they packed up the equipment that day was "But what you're proposing is a lot of work," meaning switching to whole foods instead of convenient refined ones.

I responded with, "Yeah, but Kris, dying is a lot of work. I've tried it twice." She was totally overwhelmed. She never did run the story and just about every time I called her office she was out sick.

Pat remembered that he'd had a childhood friend who was schizophrenic. This guy, we'll call him Dan, was now thirty-eight years old. He had lived in his parents' basement for the previous fifteen years. He consumed heavily sugar-laden foods, drank soft drinks and beer (which also contains added sugar) and chain-smoked. Dan spent his days watching TV, blaring rock music at seven decibels or playing Nintendo. He would sometimes get verbally abusive or violent and had generated many police actions. He had been in and out of the mental health system and had tried every drug the doctors could think of. Nothing had worked for him. Dan's family was at their wits' end.

Pat dropped by and talked to them about what we had learned about sugar. It was a slow process, but Pat has the patience of a saint. Eventually they came to trust us and so did Dan. The family paid us to take Dan in and try to detox him.

Just moving out of the basement was a significant shift for Dan. He loved the farm, he loved the animals, and he was pleased to be away from his family. The tension had been high between them all for years.

Dan had called the police a few months back and confessed to having molested a seven-year-old girl in his mother's day care about twelve years before. His family tried to convince him he was nuts and the police didn't take him seriously. They all thought it was just another one of his voices talking crazy. Dan knew it was the truth and as a born-again Christian he wanted to make restitution for his crime.

We switched him to additive-free cigarettes, got him on some of Joseph's herbs, and started him on nutritional supplements, as well as a whole foods diet. Dan had tremendous pain in his colon and a big gut to indicate his bowels were backed up. He also had the worst case of acne, from head to toe, that I have ever seen. On top of all that he had trouble sleeping.

Pat and I had moved into the Yurt after Lowell left. Patrick had taken over the master bedroom, and we made the half bedroom into a playroom with a piano in it, which was the home of Bob the turtle. Dan claimed the couch and the living room as his space. He didn't want to be too far away from the TV. He was also sharing the living room with kittens Sage, Pumpkin and Snowflake. He didn't mind their sleeping on his chest. It was a mutually satisfying arrangement for them all.

Dan heard voices, which he believed to be Satan. The voices said demeaning and crude things to him, most often in a mocking tone of voice. He would rock nervously and had many "loops" just as Lowell had. On a good day, Dan is one of the sweetest, most loving people you could ever want to meet. On a bad day, he could be a very scary being.

We had a rough beginning with Dan. Our metaphysical beliefs scared him, and he wasn't having any luck trying to shove the Bible down our throats. After a few days, we finally called a truce on the spirituality front. He was progressing so rapidly, physically and mentally, that we didn't want to scare him off. He was sleeping well, dropping weight, and his skin was showing vast improvement. Lowell had been my baby; Dan was Pat's. He deserves a ton of credit for his love and patience with Dan.

In just two weeks, Dan was down to ten addictive-free cigarettes a day from two to three packs of the regular kind. I would ration the cigarettes for him. I knew what he was going through, having had such a difficult time getting off them myself.

We had a cigarette on our sugar display table to show that cigarettes have sugar in them. Dan never touched the mountains of sugar cubes on the table, but that lone cigarette often came up missing. I finally got smart and hid it each night before going to bed. It became a standing joke.

The more Dan detoxed, the less frequently his voices would plague him. But he could still be quite anxious. It is our belief that we turn to addictions to sedate uncomfortable feelings. Consequently, when someone stops participating in the addiction those feelings are going to come to the surface.

I suspected that Dan had been sexually abused, but I didn't want to start probing yet. He had already coughed up a memory from when he was five about witnessing one of his brothers raping a neighbor girl in the very basement he lived in. I suspected there were many more memories.

Sunday morning, after about two weeks, Pat and I decided to go out for a spiritual ceremony at a farm on the outside of town. Dan was doing so well that we felt it was safe to leave for a few hours. Bad idea.

Dan called one of his friends and asked for a ride

to his parents' house. He wanted to get his stereo. We had nixed the idea because he didn't seem to have consideration for others when it came to time and volume, and we felt the dark rock and roll put him into negative loops.

When he got to his parents' house, he got anxious; that house and those people brought up old memories and feelings for him. He ate two candy bars shortly after he arrived.

When we returned from our outing, there was a phone message from Dan's mother. When we called we were told that Dan was wielding a butcher knife, and had eight Beaverton Police at bay in the basement. They were prepared to shoot him with a tranquilizer gun or worse, but had agreed to wait until we got there. They had already been there over an hour.

We sped over to Dan's house to find the living room full of cops in SWAT outfits. More cops stood on the stairs leading to the basement, having an unsuccessful conversation with a very angry, vicious Dan. I spoke with Dan's mother for a moment then headed for the basement.

Dan and I had this little game we would play. We would imitate Thurston Howell and Lovey from the old sitcom, Gilligan's Island. When I got to the head of the stairs to the basement I said, "Is that you, Thurston darling?" in my best Lovey accent.

He popped right out of his rage and cooed, "Oh, hello, Lovey" in his best Thurston Howell. We had broken his loop.

The cops at the bottom of the stairs were dumbfounded. I asked if we could come down. It was obvious that Dan was glad to see us and his demeanor had changed. I asked the officer in charge of the scene, Lieutenant Kevin O'Keefe, if we could approach Dan. Going against department policy he agreed, but first he asked Dan to set the knife to the side, which he did.

Pat and I went bounding towards Dan. We were told not to get too close. I sat right in front of him. Pat was to Dan's right. Pat talked lovingly to Dan and let him know that we were on his side. At one point I considered tackling Dan and going after the knife. When we discussed it later, Dan said that he knew I had considered that. I told him that I knew he knew. That's how close we were.

I went upstairs to negotiate with the police. Dan could not have manifested a finer set of cops. Lt. O'Keefe only cared about a nonviolent, win-win outcome. These were not the trigger-happy commandos one frequently sees on shows like Cops. They really cared about doing what was best for Dan.

Pat did a marvelous job of talking Dan down. These cops really wanted to hear that Dan had overdosed on some prescription drugs or gotten into some pot or booze. They were overwhelmed to hear that two candy bars had been the catalyst for this trauma, but it was the truth.

Before long Pat peacefully walked Dan to the living room where he sobbed and apologized to the police for all he had put them through. The sugar had run its course and we had treated him with love instead of with force. We agreed to take him for a psychiatric evaluation. If the doctor said we could take him home, we could.

We sat nervously through the hospital exam. The doctor also wanted to find some other explanation for Dan's "bump" besides sugar, but couldn't. Dan was released to us.

We made some changes after that. Dan could keep the stereo, but all the dark rock and roll had to go. We listened to peaceful, spiritual music. Dan was put in charge of brushing and feeding Sid so that he would get outside more. And we never left him alone again.

The night of the police action we decided that we should take turns watching Dan; going off to bed and leaving him alone in his overwhelm could be a mistake. Pat promptly passed out in the Yurt. I took the first shift. I rounded up all the knives in the house, wrapped them up and placed them under my pillow. Patrick was at his mother's that night so I took his bed. I figured that if I did need to sleep, I had better take the weapons with me.

I ended up staying up all night with Dan. We talked for hours. The more he talked the more he revealed about his past. We were able to identify certain painful incidents in his life when someone had said something cruel to him that had stuck in his head. As the hours rolled by, Dan began to realize that those were the voices he had attributed to Satan. It was a major breakthrough.

He also began to recognize that perhaps something sexually violent had happened to him. That thought scared him to death. One of his brothers had shared another story about the molestation of a young neighbor girl. Dan had witnessed that trauma too. The puzzle was starting to come together.

That day was the beginning of another six-day roll. Dan was to drag us through just about every agency in the state as his memories began to come back and overwhelm him. If we had known how big his mountain of pain was we probably would have opted to detox him more slowly. He was a ticking bomb.

One night he called 911 in the middle of the night. We had a second client, Tom, living with us at the time who was trying to beat his depression. By the time Tom came down to the Yurt to awaken us, the house was full of paramedics and the driveway was lined with fire trucks. Dan had passed what he thought was a bloody stool and believed that we were trying to poison him. He had too many thoughts bombarding his brain after years of heavy sedation with food, booze, cigarettes, prescription drugs and electronics; he couldn't sort it all out.

We tried to reassure him and the paramedics that it was the beets Pat had fed him for dinner the night before that he had passed. Since Dan was now calm and coherent, they had to take him to the hospital per his request.

At first the doctor treated us like idiots. After examining Dan, he rolled by us and softly confirmed "It's beets" and promptly disappeared. We took Dan home again.

A day and a half later Dan started another one of his loops. He felt we were not qualified to help him. He wanted to talk to a real counselor. We said, "Fine, you pick one and we will drive you to see him or her." Dan got on the phone and made an appointment with a counselor. I tried to be upbeat and supportive while we were waiting for the time to head out for his session. He was vile and angry with me.

I was pretty convinced that Dan had been the victim of sexual violence himself. One day he quietly admitted that I was probably right. He said he could feel a repressed memory trying to surface, but he was not ready to look at it. I encouraged him to take his time. Unfortunately, he blamed me for his problems.

I drove him to the mental health clinic. While we were waiting for his appointment, Dan began taunting and frightening a little girl in the waiting room. I barked at him and demanded he wait outside. Nobody was going to terrorize a child in my presence. Outside he went. Finally, the therapist came to get Dan. After a few minutes he sent Dan back out to have a cigarette and asked to speak with me. The man looked sincerely scared. He told me that Dan had talked about murdering Pat and me. He was genuinely afraid for me but indicated that there was nothing he could do. He walked me to the parking lot and watched as I got back in the truck with this very angry, dangerous guy.

I was scared. My third degree black-belt skills don't serve me well when I am strapped in behind the wheel in rush-hour traffic. I said, "Okay, Dan, what are we going to do?"

"Take me to my parents' house," he barked.

"No, you know I can't do that. You promised the police you would stay away from there. Your choices are to come back to the farm with me and do what you committed to do, or we can go to the police station and you can play games with them. What do you want to do?"

He cockily remarked, "Okay, let's go to the police station."

"Fine with me," I snipped and started to drive. As soon as we got deep in rush-hour traffic he sat up on the edge of his seat, got right in my face with a hideous grin, and told me that he was going to murder me in my sleep. I drove, ready to maneuver the truck off the road at the slightest sign of violence.

When we arrived at the Beaverton police station I parked the truck and said, "Hey, go piss these guys off." Dan got out of the truck and headed inside to do his thing. In general he hated the police. Lt. O'Keefe was the only cop he had ever warmed up to.

Dan was being a pain in the ass, but fortunately (or not, this particular day) there is no law prohibiting being a jerk. I went in and told the officer who was there that Dan had told a counselor that he was going to murder Pat and me and that he had threatened to murder me in my sleep on the way over. They told me there was nothing they could do. Dan was outside smoking. I went to the pay phone and called Pat. I hadn't slept in days and couldn't handle any more. I asked Pat to come take over.

Pat arrived with one of Dan's brothers. I took off in the truck and went home to bed. While Pat and Dan's brother were busy speaking with the police, Dan quietly walked away from the police station and headed to his family's home, a mile away. That was the beginning of the next round with the police.

Suffice it to say, this story goes on and on. Dan continued to generate police actions and eventually wound up in the state mental hospital. Lt. O'Keefe worked with us tirelessly, but the system really isn't set up for prevention. We had to goad Dan into threatening a cop so that he wouldn't have to commit a more serious crime to get help. We couldn't handle him anymore.

His psychiatrist at the state mental hospital spoke with us. She had been doing some studies on food to see if there was something that was setting people off. She hadn't considered the sugar but invited us to send her information. She ordered special whole foods for Dan and allowed us to ship him vitamins and minerals. She could see that he did well when he ate whole foods and went downhill when he got into the sugar. Finally, somebody was listening.

We showed up at every court date and stood behind Dan, continuing to show him love. Dan's willingness to peek at his pain and our boldness to take him on changed his life forever.

After Dan left we went into another emotional nosedive. We were up to our eyeballs in debt and few people wanted to hear the truth about sugar. The landowners, Sydney and Ron Willett, were now considering selling the farm. Our attorney, Kyle Rotenberg, had offered to purchase the land, if it ever came up for sale, and give us an opportunity to develop it into a teaching facility for holistic and sustainable technologies. It was a very valuable property for its prime location in Beaverton, Oregon, the home of Nike, Intel and Tektronics, to name a few.

We had met a neat couple, Tom Hudson and Lucia

Soppe. They had a healing practice and were helping us tackle our emotional issues and promote our business. They believed wholeheartedly in our mission to educate people about food and eventually to build communities around sacred energy gardens, but they weren't too sure about our approach.

One day they recommended that we consider giving up the "sugar thing" and just talk to people about whole foods. We were pretty low that day. We didn't want to believe that we had to "sugarcoat" our message in order to get people's attention. We decided to take the day off and go see a movie. We hadn't spent ten cents or a single afternoon on ourselves in six months. We needed a break.

By this time we didn't have a vehicle anymore. Our truck had died, and I had long since lost my Neon to the loan sharks. Pioneering a new concept is never easy, especially when it smacks into the biggest addiction on the planet. We walked to the bus stop and headed off for an afternoon matinee.

We decided to see Trial and Error, which starred Michael Richards and Jeff Daniels. It looked like a fun comedy. It turned out that the movie revolves around a trial where they use the infamous "Twinkie Defense" to attempt to get a guilty client off. There actually was a trial in San Francisco in 1981 where a man had committed a double homicide. One of the victims was the mayor of San Francisco. His lawyers had gotten the killer, Dan White, a reduced sentence because they showed a long pattern of depression that was directly linked to his junk food consumption. He was high on Twinkies at the time of the murders. It was not a popular verdict at the time.

Trial and Error was making fun of the Twinkie defense. Nonetheless, they were getting the information out. In one scene they put up a chart with the molecular structure of sugar and the molecular structure of cocaine. The next chart compared chocolate to screamed and hooted as the rest of the sparse audience quietly ate their M&M's and drank their giant tumblers of liquid sugar. We considered it an act of God that of all the available movies we had chosen this one. We had to forge on.

Pat and I have committed our lives to speaking out about the dangers of this widely loved, mind-altering substance. Consuming it nearly killed us; talking about it might just finish the job.

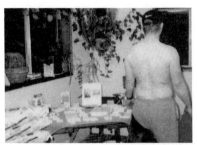

Dan in front of the sugar display.

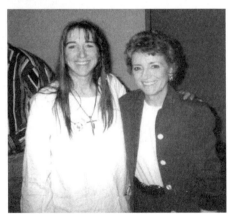

Me and Reverend Mary during my hemp tent phase.

FOOD FOR THOUGHT...

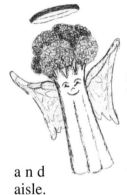

The bottom line is that we have to get back to balance. We are way out of line on the sugar thing. How many people do you know who eat 150 pounds of brown rice or broccoli each year. The produce departments of our grocery stores get smaller and smaller a n d the refined carbohydrates are on every aisle.

We worked with a number of different individuals with varying challenges, like Sal, who was blind and came to live with us for a weekend. By Sunday he was running around, gleefully announcing, "I'm so happy!"

A child with ADHD stayed with us for ten days and pulled out of her destructive behaviors. Another autistic kid found his way to us. Everybody improved on a diet of whole foods, safety and extra helpings of love and acceptance. Those, like Lowell, who were willing to face their old "stuff" experienced some quantum leaps. It was more confirmation for our theory that we are what we eat, as well as what we believe.

JUST FOR FUN...

Reverend Mary told us this story the day we went to talk to her about serving sugar at her church. I love Mary. Her cable ministry has touched millions of lives around the world.

A woman with a sick child went to great lengths to get an audience with Ghandi. She had waited long and traveled far. When she finally got the master's ear, she asked him to tell her son to stop eating sugar. The Mahatma said, "Come back in two weeks."

She waited the two weeks, traveled the long distance to her meeting, and approached the Great One again.

"You said if I came back in two weeks you would tell my son to quit eating sugar," the woman pleaded.

Ghandi turned to the child and said, "Don't eat sugar."

The woman was pleased but perplexed. She asked, "How come you made me wait two weeks to tell him that?"

"Because, Madame, two weeks ago I was still eating sugar."

.

TRAVEL TALES

It has been two and a half years since I wrote the previous chapter of this book. And the final chapter has been rewritten three times in that period. No matter how many raves I received I just couldn't seem to raise the rest of the capital I needed to publish this book. I finally realized that it wasn't funded or on the market yet because it wasn't finished.

Knowing how I live my life you can imagine how much has happened since I last wrote. These last three chapters reflect a lifetime of spiritual growth acquired in two and a half years. If you have been shocked by my life thus far, hold on! I have been living in fast-forward.

Pat and I lost the farm. The owner, Sidney Willett, did not honor the long-standing agreement to give Pat the first right of refusal that her banker-father, Bob Hazen, had promised him for fifteen years. Even though we had backers who had committed to help us buy the property, we never stood a chance against the owners, the developers and the county. Fourteen cats, Bob the turtle, and Pat and I became homeless, and the bulldozers destroyed our little piece of heaven. Our horse Sid and Scooby the dog fared better. They ended up with wonderful homes and loving families.

After losing the farm, I put out a flyer announcing, "Have Yurt Will Travel." We were looking for a family willing to pay to have us in their backyard, growing and serving sacred foods for their health and enlightenment. The press was quite interested, but we never found any takers.

Friends and family passed us around as we struggled to get on our feet. We weren't particularly welcome anywhere we stayed because of our strict diet and constant sermons about sugar. Even when we gave up the evangelism, we still weren't welcome. We were beginning to recognize that most people have a lot of shame and guilt about the way they eat and feed their kids. It was easier to beat up the messengers than change.

But we knew we had a key solution to many health and psychiatric problems, as well as a gateway to heaven. And so we flew to Richmond, Virginia, with twenty-five dollars in our pocket and a beautiful sixty-page, four-color business plan to meet with an investment company. They were interested in helping us find funding for our "Celebrity Sugar Detox Center."

On the flight out, Pat and I had made quite a scene as we boarded the plane. I was hauling the sugar display I had made: six twenty-five-pound bags of sugar, drained, stuffed, glued together and shellacked, with a handle on the side — a physical representation of this country's annual per capita consumption of refined sugar. I had to carry it over my head to get down the narrow aisle to where the flight attendant was to stow it in the rear of the aircraft.

We settled comfortably into our seats, declining the headphones for the movie because we didn't have enough money. When the lights dimmed and the movie came on we roared with excitement over the "silent" film we were about to view again. We considered it another act of God as Trial and Error (the anti-sugar movie

I spoke of in the last chapter) played to a sleepy audience of travelers.

The Austrian Baron who owned the investment company turned out to be quite the character. He dressed like Mickey Rooney on a golf outing, but had a very commanding presence for a man of five-foot-nothing. He also made good copy when he graced the front page of USA Today a few weeks later for forty-nine years of fraud. Fortunately, we hadn't given him any money, even though our camp had been willing to ante up.

We then went on to Atlanta to meet with an investment broker with whom I had developed a long-standing relationship by phone. I had helped him close an important deal so he was hosting us as a thank you for my business savvy. Alan was a recovered alcoholic who was now a hard-core sugar junkie. While we were staying with him he fell off the wagon and generated a very lively police action. Alan tried to have us arrested. Instead the police escorted him out of his own home and applauded us for not letting him drive drunk.

We also found our way onto CNN's Talk Back Live while in Atlanta. We overwhelmed every producer, director and host who didn't move fast enough. We would patiently wait in line each day in the lobby of the CNN building where the show was taped. We would anxiously raise our hands to comment whenever they allowed the audience to participate. No matter what the topic of the day was, we would find a way to question the guest about toxic foods. During commercials we would summon the host or a producer and attempt to recruit them for the mission. After a few days they learned how to scan the audience without ever acknowledging us. America, for the most part, apparently wasn't ready to face its sugar addiction yet.

This next traveling story is a bit out of sequence. I

Letters From Heaven, but it really belongs here. This is my favorite adventure to date. It began the last week of August 1999.

In my dream I was traveling with Oprah as a member of a dance troupe she was sponsoring. Although we had been on the road together for a while I had not gotten the opportunity to actually talk with Oprah. Finally, I see her seated alone in a booth at the restaurant we had taken over for dinner. Swiftly, I slid in next to her and quizzed, "Oprah, hasn't anyone ever talked to you about the connection between food and spirituality?"

She softly whispered, "No."

"Forget about your weight, forget about your health, wouldn't you like to be closer to God?" I probed.

Oprah looked me square in the eyes with genuine interest and said, "Tell me more."

I woke up exhilarated! I had been plotting a pilgrimage to Chicago to hunt Oprah for weeks. This was a good omen, even though I had no money and no plan yet on how to get to Chicago, get into the studios, or get her attention. Meeting Phil Donohue had only taken a few hours; Oprah, no doubt, would require a bigger effort.

I packed, filled my water bottle and grabbed Henry. (Henry was an adorable pink stuffed monkey I had recently found abandoned in a barn. This darn little monkey really had a personality that makes fully grown folks go gaga. Henry felt like a piece of myself that I had abandoned in childhood. I invited that part of me home by nurturing Henry.)

I had less than a dollar in change in my pocket and I hadn't eaten. "Oh well," I thought, "God will provide." As that thought drifted through me I put my very heavy pack down on the side of the road. As I set it down

I noticed a blackberry bush pregnant with fruit, "Thank you, God," I announced as I dined.

I am a very seasoned hitchhiker. I knew that I could get to Chicago fairly effortlessly if I could just get the twenty-five miles or so to the truck stop on Interstate 5 (The major freeway that runs through Portland, Oregon). However, I was on a small farm road a ways from town and the prospects looked bleak.

After twenty minutes or so I declared, "Okay, God, if I am supposed to go to Chicago, then I will leave it in your hands to get me a ride." Within moments I arrived at the truck stop. I was committed now; it was time to start formulating a plan. I plopped down in the phone room because that's where the truckers usually hang out, but there was no one at any of the eight phone stations. The television caught my eye though; the Chicago Bears were plowing their way down the field. "Okay, God, I get it. I'm going!"

An instant later a man came in, sat down and picked up the phone. I heard him tell the person on the other end of the line that he had a load out to Chicago in the morning. When he hung up the phone I asked, "Do you believe in God?"

"Of course!" he replied, almost indignant that I had asked.

"Well, I sat down here looking for a ride to Chicago and I heard you say that you have a load going there in the morning. Will you take me?" He explained that his load was going to Chicago but that he would probably get turned around in Salt Lake. But maybe the next driver would take me to Chicago. I said, "Perfect. I can get anywhere in the country from Salt Lake." John Lawrence agreed to take me at least as far as Salt Lake and told me where and when to find him in the morning.

John turned out to be a lot of fun. We talked, laughed and listened to the blues for a day and a half. He didn't get turned around in Salt Lake, so we continued east. At one point I remember John looking at me and saying, "I get the Henry thing. He's got quite a spirit to him." Little Henry, the world's first traveling Evangelist monkey – pink no less! John was a member of the ministry by now. He had seen all the pictures, my book, heard the rap, and was chanting "Oprah" with me as we passed each mile marker.

John got the word that he would swap his load with a trucker named Roderick, in Cheyenne. Roderick rolled into the truck stop shortly after dark. I knew that he was good people immediately, because he had stuffed animals in the window of his cab. Finally, some company for Henry! Roderick agreed to take me on to Chicago but needed to sleep for six hours or so first. John and I watched a movie in his cab before I crawled into the top bunk of Roderick's truck for a toasty nap. Yes, trucks now have TVs, VCRs, stereos and sometimes refrigerators and microwaves — the Rolls Royce of travel for a hitchhiker.

Roderick Moore was big and black. I only had a two-minute conversation with him before crawling into his truck to go to sleep for the night, but I felt totally safe. My plan had been to get out and get a fresh ride every time a trucker I was traveling with stopped to sleep. But Roderick was so much fun that I didn't want to get out. I spent the next three days with him. We had eleven hundred miles of cornfields to look at so we passed the hours telling stories. He had some dandies!

One night I woke up in the middle of the night and Henry was gone. I started to panic but realized that he couldn't have gotten far in the cab of this truck. Finally, out of curiosity, I peeked down from my bunk at Roderick sleeping below. There was Henry perched happily next to Roderick. It was decidedly a Kodak moment.

We rolled into a suburb of Chicago about happy hour on Thursday afternoon — eighty hours after I had left Portland. Roderick had to deliver in the morning and promised to help me get downtown after he dropped his load. We went to a local bar he frequented when in the area. I was ready to start hunting Oprah and asked for a phone book. The litany from the locals was, "You'll never get in to see Oprah. You have to be somebody, know somebody or wait months for tickets." Roderick knew me well by now. He sipped his beer and laughed as he assured them that I would find a way.

I called Oprah's company, Harpo Productions. The operator in charge of tickets jumped right into the "You'll never get in at this late date" litany. She didn't seem to have any sympathy for my story. But then — we had what I call a "God moment."

She said, "You go to the concierge at the hotel you're staying at and see if they can get you some tickets." (Like I had hitchhiked cross-country to stay at the Hilton!) But I felt it when she said it. "That's it! That's how God is going to get me into that studio." Now I had a plan.

Roderick and I got some food for dinner and headed over to Blockbuster to rent a movie. We parked the truck in the parking lot of a grocery store so we could use the bathroom and get supplies as we laughed and cried over "Patch Adams." (For the record. Roderick was a happily married man. He reached out to me as a friend he respected. There was nothing more between us.)

After one of my bathroom breaks I returned to the truck to find a Chicago cop parked in front of it. The officer was finishing up some paperwork. I told him my tale expecting a sermon on the dangers of hitchhiking. Instead he proclaimed, "God bless you, lady, we need more people like you!" I gave him an article about our vision of curbing violence in the schools and headed back to the truck.

The next morning we waited while the trailer was

unloaded and reloaded. Although only a year older than I, Roderick was becoming an overprotective father who didn't want to set me loose on the streets of Chicago. But the time had come.

We parked the truck and walked about a mile to the train station. Roderick was in a panic the whole way. "Are you sure you want to do this? I can get you a ride back home."

"Roderick, I'm committed now, I have to do this. Don't worry, I'll be okay. God is with me." He swapped me a ten-dollar bill for a one then had me buy him a Coke with a twenty and let me keep the change. He was getting quite militant now. "I'm gonna call Oprah and make sure they let you in! You call me. You let me know what happened."

I assured him I would as he hugged me good-bye. I felt the "ouch" of parting with a friend I might never see again. (Thanks, Roderick, you're a gem!) Now I was about to really test my faith. I had three hours till sundown, didn't know a soul in Chicago, hadn't been there in thirty years and had $57 left to my name. (John had squeezed a twenty in my palm before we parted. Patrick, still my ever-loyal partner in this ministry about food, had picked up an odd job and wired me $80, and, of course, there was Roderick's generosity – thank you, God!) Here we go...

I thought that Oprah housed her guests at the Embassy Suites so I headed there. It would be about a mile walk from where the train had dumped me down-town. I got lots of attention as I bounced down the streets with Henry hanging out of my pack.

I walked into the Embassy Suites, put my pack down on the floor and approached the concierge's desk. The man behind the desk was an enormous black man wearing a nametag that read "Rodrick."

I sat down at his desk and said, "I can't believe that your name is Rodrick!" He smiled.

"I work for God. I hitchhiked 2100 miles to talk to Oprah about the connection between food and spirituality. The people at her studios tell me that my only shot at getting in is to suck up to a concierge, so I am sucking up." He smiled again. Rodrick explained that Oprah only taped on Tuesdays, Wednesdays and Thursdays. He was indicating that I was out of luck until Tuesday.

"Doesn't matter to me. I'm not leaving until I meet her." He said that they call the studios at 2pm on Monday to inquire about tickets for Tuesday. He made a note in his day planner to call on Monday and another note for Tuesday in case I didn't get in first try. He told me to call about 2:30 on Monday. With tears in my eyes I shook his hand and said, "God bless you."

I carried my pack over the to bellman's desk. For a two-dollar tip I could stow it while I cruised Chicago looking for a home for the next four days. My plan was to sit in one bar or another and tell my story until somebody said, "Gee, you can stay at my house for the weekend." (Fortunately, I am an attractive woman in my early forties, with personality and savvy. It was a reasonable plan.)

Vince Winters and his three roommates opened their home to me. Although I didn't see much of them, they treated me like family. (Thanks Vince, John, Kevin and Tim!) On Monday I nervously called the Embassy Suites at 2:30. I got a different concierge this time. Rodrick was off for the next two days. This foreign-sounding woman said that Oprah wasn't taping on Tuesday. (Actually, I found out later that Oprah taped a show on food addiction that day.) The concierge told me to call back the next day. I went to see her in person instead. I was concerned that she wasn't going to do this for me as she kept asking if I had checked in yet.

Vince had given me a ride downtown and lent me

his umbrella. I walked around in the pouring rain for some time. I was consumed with fear. I kept repeating my, "God is more powerful than a concierge, than Harpo studios, than Oprah" mantra, but it wasn't sinking in.

At 2:30 I entered the Embassy Suites. The concierge was not at her desk. I felt a sense of panic. I went upstairs to the lounge area that overlooked the lobby. I threw a dime in the fountain and said a prayer. I sat down and set out to conquer my fear. "Look, Denise, you better get over this quick! You create your own reality and you are about to create a disaster. God is more powerful than a concierge is. God is more powerful than Harpo studios. God is more powerful than Oprah. Now leave it in God's hands and have faith!" I leaned over the rail and observed that the concierge had returned to her desk. It must be time, I thought.

I headed down the stairs trying to deny the fear I still felt. "God is more powerful..." I stood nervously in front of her desk and peeped, "Any luck?"

"Yes. You need to be there between eleven and twelve in the morning. They are taping a show and a half tomorrow so you'll have to plan to be there all afternoon."

Mission accomplished! I knew that once I was in the same room with Oprah I could tell her my story. I was in! I got the rest of the information I needed, blessed the concierge with tear-filled eyes and headed out into the rain. I walked the streets and cried with joy for an hour before burning up the remainder of my phone card calling home. Twenty hours to Oprah.

Wednesday I set out my only dress and fluffed Henry's furry little head. I wanted us to look our best for the occasion. I packed carefully. I had one pile to give to Oprah, which included a copy of my bound manuscript, the articles that had been written about Pat and me, and a CD of Mark Olmstead's, a performer who had recently joined the mission. I had a pile of laminated blown-up photos of our sacred energy gardens to show the folks in the audience.

Roommate John drove me downtown to the studios. The line was already snaking around the building. I joined the crowd with Henry peeking out of my purse. While waiting to get into the studio I bonded with a very handsome couple from the suburbs of Chicago, Bob and Kathleen Jones. They were quite supportive of my mission and curious to see how I was going to get Oprah's attention.

Security took my gifts for Oprah and assured me that she would receive them. They also took my day planner, my coat, pictures, water bottle and even Henry. I felt a twinge of fear as I watched Henry disappear into the security area. All I had was a little ticket with a number on it. What if somebody stole Henry? I noted that it was profound that Henry and the concierge were the things that had brought up fear in me, whereas I had put my life on the line to travel cross-country on foot without giving it a thought.

Once inside the building all two hundred of us audience members were crammed into a tiny room that had a table full of sugary treats and beverages in the middle. I found a small bottle of water on the other side of the room, chatted with Bob and Kathleen about the junk food spread, and got in line for the bathroom.

Before long, we were called into the studio. We could sit wherever we wanted. I found one lone seat by a walkway. It turned out that just on the other side of the railing from my seat was where the producers and directors stood and where Oprah and the guests would be coming out. I smiled to myself, as it appeared that divine intervention was obviously still orchestrating this adventure.

A charismatic young black man with a microphone took the stage to warm up the audience. He told us that the first taping was about dysfunctional families that weren't getting along. After chatting some about the second show we would be taping and leading us in a few cheers to get the energy rolling, the man with the microphone asked if we had any questions. I leapt to my feet.

"I hitchhiked 2100 miles to see Oprah. Am I going to be able to meet her, shake her hand, look her in the eye?"

"Wow!" he responded. "You must really like the show."

"I do."

"Well, sometimes she greets the audience after the show, but not always. But you can make a comment during a commercial or something."

I was very relaxed now, no fear. I knew that my wild personality would get Oprah's attention. I just had to choose my moment.

The man with the mike also reminded us that Oprah had started teaching at the university the night before. (She had been all over the local news. They were now calling her "Professor Winfrey." Chicago is so proud of Oprah.) Following a grand introduction and thunderous applause, Oprah walked by me and into the spotlight.

The show was a very emotional one. Some of the guests were sobbing and the expert, Mark Bryan, who was trying to get them through this, was working hard. I felt that these guests deserved the attention right now so I sat quietly for the first forty minutes. About the fifth commercial I decided to make my move.

The studio was set up like a theatre. The stage was a small platform in the middle of the room, raised a few inches, surrounded by cameras and lights, with four plain chairs on it where Oprah, Mark and the two guests were seated. The audience chairs were in a semicircle on tiers. My seat was about five rows up from the stage.

I headed towards the bathroom. After passing the

last camera I took a sharp right turn with the intention of walking up onto the stage and chatting with Oprah. A tall security man grabbed me. I leaned around him, looked at Oprah, who was looking right at me from about fifteen feet away, and said loudly, "I just want to tell her that I hitchhiked 2100 miles to give her a message."

Oprah said, "What's the message?" The security man released me. I now had Oprah's ear as well as the attention of the other two hundred people in the room.

"I work for God. I hitchhiked 2100 miles after having a dream about you, to give you a message."

"What's the message?" she repeated.

"There is a connection between food and spirituality. I nearly died from sixteen years of bulimia, and what I have learned in my recovery is that food is part of the spiritual journey. I've written a book about my recovery. There is a copy along with some other materials in the package I left for you."

As she squirmed in her chair, she jokingly said, "Is there any food in the package, some cheesecake or something?"

"No, and there wasn't any food in what you served us upstairs, either."

"2100 miles. Where are you from?"

"Portland, Oregon."

She was quite serious now, leaning forward in her chair. "Isn't hitchhiking dangerous?"

"Yes, but you're not an easy gal to get to. After eight years of writing to your production company I finally decided that I had to come. I probably have the only information about food that you haven't heard." Oprah was speechless. It was time for the commercial to end so I quietly headed back to my seat.

During the next commercial I shouted out, "So, Professor, how'd it go?"

Oprah talked about how scared and intimidated

she had been at first until she realized that these high-powered business people who were taking her leadership course were just people. She had apparently relaxed into her new role with great pleasure. (Go, Oprah!)

During the next commercial she talked about the fact that she wasn't a control freak, it's just that she's always right. It was a struggle to figure out whether she was kidding or not. We laughed nervously throughout her soliloquy which also included the information that she and Stedman own a farm in Indiana a few hours away. My little sacred-energy-farming brain started clicking away.

The first show ended and Oprah went off to her dressing room to change. We had each received a copy of Mark Bryan's book, Codes of Love, as a gift. When he got up to sign autographs he came straight to me, shook my hand vigorously and pronounced, "Congratulations, and good luck with your book!" I basked in the validation for a moment. (Thanks, Mark, I love your book!)

The set was rearranged, the guests recycled, and Oprah came out in a hot new outfit. This next show was going to be an emotional one too. During the first commercial, Oprah asked one of the camera people if he remembered the first show they had taped that day. (They had shot one before the two I witnessed.) He swiftly gave her the information. She chuckled, "It's a good thing you knew. I was going to bet you a hundred dollars you wouldn't."

"Pretty easy gamble when you're always right," I bellowed. She didn't like that. I felt it from across the room. "That was stupid, Denise," I chastised myself. I committed to keeping my mouth shut the rest of the show.

When it was over, Oprah hugged the guests and then headed for the exit that led to her dressing room. I was in a daze. I awoke realizing that she was high-fiving the people in front of me on her way out of the studio. I threw my hand out as an afterthought. When she got to me she grabbed my hand and pulled me towards her. She peered deep into my eyes as if to say, "Who are you lady?" I smiled lovingly at her.

I retrieved Henry and my things and hit the pavement. I was down to a few dollars, exhausted and anxious to get home. I had been praying that Oprah or one of the audience members would be moved to help me. No deal. My return trip took a lot more effort as I didn't choose to sleep or hang. I can't even remember all the sweet travelers and truckers that graced my trip home, but I am grateful for each one of them. I stepped back onto Portland soil exactly fifty hours after I left Chicago. Suffice it to say, my trip home was as magical as my trip out. Spirit was with me every step of the way.

Oprah hasn't called or responded to my letters, but that thirteen days and 4200 miles was the most valuable experience of my life to date. I learned how to "let go and let God." I had a few fears along the way, but I acknowledged them and kept moving. I never let them stop me.

As for Oprah, it is my belief that we each create our own reality. She manifested me to barge into her life with this information the day after she taped a show on food addiction — admittedly her greatest inadequacy. What she does with the information I brought her is her business. My job was to tell her.

I had four names on my hit list, movers and shakers I wanted to recruit for the mission. The first person was Mike Mikesell, the vice president of Albertina Kerr. You'll read about how that turned out in the next chapter. The second was Reverend Mary Manin Morrissey, who has a global New-Thought ministry. Mary has recently started including information about food and health in her sermons. Oprah makes three down. I believe that before long she will join the mission.

As for the fourth name on my list: White House security is going to be a bear, but Henry and I will find a way! (Well, Bill Clinton has left office since I originally wrote this, so I guess a pilgrimage to Harlem is in order.)

FOOD FOR THOUGHT...

When I set out to write Eating My Way to Heaven, my dream was to educate people about the effect food has on us physically, mentally and spiritually. I hope that I have managed to impart some useful information on that front. In the four years since I started this book, though, I have learned a lot and shifted my thinking somewhat.

I believe that the ability to have an emotion is the greatest gift God has given us humans. And facing our emotions is the hardest work there is. I am no longer so focused on food as being the root of our problems. I now see that there are all kinds of ways to run away from the work that we came here to do. Food addiction is just one of many distractions. We can sedate our emotions with food, drugs, alcohol, coffee and/or cigarettes, or escape them through television, music, the Internet, sex or spending money, to name a few.

It is my belief that there is only one thing we can take with us when we leave this world — the spiritual growth we have attained in this lifetime. We know for sure that we can't take our stuff or our money. So why do we put such a high value on these things and so little value on feeling and experiencing?

I literally ate my way to heaven on Earth. But I now realize that going broke was one of the ingredients

I plan to amass a lot of wealth through my writing and my ventures in this lifetime. But you won't find my money sitting in a bank. I plan to share it with those with less and those seeking to make the planet a better place. Working together as a people we can learn to embrace our emotions and grow. That is the basis of true wealth for me.

JUST FOR FUN...

Just for fun...Speaking of food and God...Mother Theresa died and went to heaven. God greets her at the Pearly Gates.

"Be Thou hungry, Mother Theresa?" asks God.

"I could eat," Mother Theresa replies.

So God opens a can of tuna and reaches for a chunk of rye bread and they share it. While eating this humble meal, Mother Theresa looks down into Hell and sees the inhabitants devouring huge steaks, lobsters, pheasants, pastries and wines. Curious, but deeply trusting, she remains quiet.

The next day God again invites her to join him for a meal. Again, it is tuna and rye bread. Once again, Mother Theresa can see the denizens of Hell enjoying caviar, champagne, lamb, truffles, and chocolates. Still she says nothing.

The following day, mealtime arrives and another can of tuna is opened. She can't contain herself any longer. Meekly, she says, "God, I am grateful to be in heaven with you as a reward for the pious obedient life I led. But here in heaven all I get to eat is tuna and a piece of rye bread. In the Other Place they eat like emperors and kings. I just don't understand."

God sighs, "Let's be honest. For just two people, does it pay to cook?"

CIRCLES OF LOVE

One day, shortly before we lost the farm, I was hitchhiking home. A distinguished looking gentleman picked me up. On the way to the farm I gave him "the rap." It turned out that he was the Vice President of Albertina Kerr, the largest nonprofit in Oregon that works with abused children. Upon meeting Pat and touring the farm, Mike Mikesell declared, "Now this is how you treat children."

After meeting us, Mike had tried to implement a program like ours at their facility, but couldn't get the powers-that-be of Albertina Kerr to go for it. They have three psychiatrists on board who each pulls down a hefty salary for medicating children into submission. They didn't want to consider that there was a more humane way.

Pat just couldn't let go of the idea that the children at Albertina Kerr deserved love and good food more than locked doors and Ritalin. He hounded Dr. Mikesell until he finally brought us in the back door on a small grant. In the pouring rain of January 1998 we broke ground on the first of our three sacred energy gardens at Albertina Kerr in Gresham, Oregon.

We wanted to make it fun and interesting for the kids, so we dug round gardens. Twenty-five hundred square feet each, they looked like alien-generated crop circles.

We set out to make the first circle look like the Mayan calendar, which has twenty-eight spokes to it. (Coincidentally, so did the ceiling of our Yurt, which we moved onto the Albertina Kerr property.) We realized that the pathways would take up too much space so we just started digging and decided to see what we could come up with. We ended up with twenty-two individual plots in a divine pattern. Two days later a member of the Kerr staff showed up with the roster of children who would be working in the garden. There were twenty-two lucky names on the list!

We dug the second circle in a spiral and planted it all in corn so the kids could just run wild through it like a magical maze. The third circle had quadrants that Pat made up as he went along. Our friend Tom helped with the digging as a means of working his way out of depression. He really loved the kids. They loved him and his dog, Theo, and helped him rekindle a desire to live.

The kids were only allowed to participate in the garden for one hour, once a week. They helped to till, plant, weed and water their beds. My mother had sent darling nametags for each child that we laminated and posted at the end of each plot. The children excitedly dragged their families to the garden (if they were lucky enough to have a family, or one that would visit).

The pyramids are believed to have special powers due, in part, to the synergy of geometry and nature working together. The same seemed to be true of our crop circles; thus we called them "Sacred Energy Gardens." What happened to the plants in those gardens was nothing short of miraculous. Mother Nature gifted these deeply unhappy children with beets the size of grapefruits, sunflowers too big for their stalks, peas as sweet as candy and flowers that glowed and danced in the breeze.

Our encounters with the children were so heart-warming that our difficult circumstances seemed worth it. We had been allowed to set up our Yurt behind the maintenance shop. The laborers who worked there were great guys who loved what we were doing and were very supportive.

Albertina Kerr's philosophy seemed to be to keep the children medicated so that they don't have an emotion that might spur them to become suicidal. And don't show them too much affection or they will be devastated when they leave. You couldn't hug them (except for an occasional side hug) and it was forbidden to say "I love you" or talk about God, no matter how much these lonely children pleaded for such support. The only way to get around the rules was with a wheelbarrow and permission to head to the compost pile.

Lots of affection and discussions about spirit took place on those journeys to retrieve some soil. We showed the children more genuine love than the rules allowed. Consequently, the kids went wild every time we crossed the compound, which didn't endear us to the psychiatrists one bit.

The hardest part about living there was watching the daily routines of these young kids. Most of them had been horribly abused or abandoned, and a few had committed criminal acts in their rage and pain. They were locked up, indoors, almost twenty-three hours a day. They were heavily medicated and fed high-sugar, high-carbohydrate diets. They were treated like robots, marched single file from place to place, then tied facedown on a table in a cell-like room if their rage ever seeped out and annoyed anyone.

I was about to have a nervous breakdown from heartache, observing all this. We knew the end of our association with Albertina Kerr was near, though, after we witnessed a very disturbing incident in the garden one day.

Little Jimmy (I've changed his name to protect him) came to the garden with his counselor. Pat and I and one other child were also there. Jimmy wanted to work in the spiral garden with me, but his counselor insisted that he work with her in the third circle. She wasn't really working with him though. She was just doing her own thing. It was obvious to me that Jimmy craved some freedom of choice and more attention. When he didn't get it, he threw a tantrum. He was furiously pulling potato plants up by the roots. I politely said, "Jimmy, please don't do that."

Before he could react, his 150-pound counselor jumped him. Jimmy was eight or nine years old and weighed about 60 pounds soaking wet. He looked like a cherub-faced child from a cereal commercial, with big bright eyes and a splash of freckles on his nose. The counselor started dragging him out of the potatoes, reprimanding him for his behavior. The more physical she became, the louder he screamed. She straddled his back, put him in a police hold with his face in the dirt, and pulled his little legs up tightly towards his bottom. When Jimmy screamed louder she sent the other child to get his psychiatrist.

Pat and I were not allowed to interfere with the staff. All we could do was observe in horror as the counselor and the psychiatrist hauled this poor child out of the garden like a hardened criminal in a state-sanctioned police hold, as per the foundation's rules. We were confident that a little love and attention would have prevented the whole incident. I went to Mike Mikesell and discussed my feelings about what had happened. Mike was continually torn between his loyalty to the foundation and his dedication to what we were doing. He agreed that perhaps there could have been a better way to handle Jimmy that day.

Before long we were told that we would be hosting a harvest party for the children on September 19th and that our services would no longer be needed. They were selling the land, or leasing it, or something, and wouldn't be able to accommodate our project the following year.

The harvest party was bittersweet for us. The children were allowed a fair level of frenzy that day. They each received a plastic garbage bag and were invited to take whatever they wanted from their own plots and whatever they could negotiate from someone else's. The kids were so excited. It was like Halloween. The exhilarating thing was that they were vying for potatoes, beets and peas, instead of Snickers, Hershey bars and lollipops.

Albertina Kerr brought some other very challenged children and adults to the garden that day, and a cadre of reporters and photographers to document the event. Although we weren't invited to continue our project, they slapped us all over the cover and back of their annual report that year, as well as numerous pages in-between. They didn't want to admit that our program (which cost them $20,000 of their $22,000,000 budget) was more effective than theirs, but they did recognize it as a great tool for soliciting donations. The generous donors were never told that this program, which the children adored, had been discontinued.

We have always been grateful for Dr. Mikesell; so were the children of Albertina Kerr.

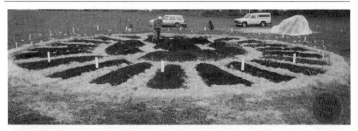

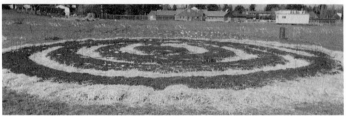

This is two of the three circle gardens we built with the children of Albertina Kerr.

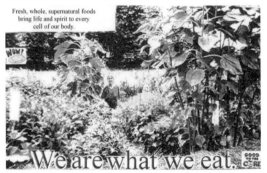

This is two of the above plots halfway through the summer. This is SuPRANAtural™ food!

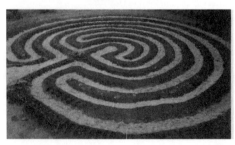

This is a onehalf acre Labrinth Garden that we built in Hubbard, Oregon.

FOOD FOR THOUGHT...

There are agencies like Albertina Kerr in every state. They honestly believe that they are rendering a much-needed service and are doing right by the children. Indeed, most of the children were better off in the hands of the Albertina Kerr professionals than they were at home. But we feel there is much room for evolution in the way they administer treatment for the children in their care. It will never happen, though, unless we all commit to stop looking the other way and do something. Check out what is being done for the "forgotten" children in your state and get involved. You will be richly rewarded. I promise!

JUST FOR FUN

The children of Albertina Kerr taught us a thing or two about hope and faith. I fell in love with one of the kids whom I thought I might adopt one day, if they didn't release him to his grandmother, as he and she wished. (They eventually did. Thank you, God. I hear he is quite happy.) Little Mike was an amazing being. He opened my heart considerably.

Prior to his first day in the garden, he had been reading a science fiction (or not) book about these beings from another planet that came to Earth and built circular gardens. Needless to say, he was wide-eyed when he first stepped foot in our Eden. Mike and I bonded right away. He was a very spiritual child and we talked about God every chance we got to slip away to the compost pile.

It seems that Mike had a little girlfriend named Rosie. He decided that he wanted a dozen roses to take to her, so he asked me to get a rose bush that we could plant. I explained to him, "Gee, Mike, rose bushes are kind of spendy. We could buy a lot of produce seeds for the price of one rose bush."

"Well," he responded matter-of-factly, "I guess you'll just have to negotiate." Mike was ten years old but had the communication skills of an adult. So I set out to sweet-talk the owner of the nursery to gift us with a rose bush for Mike. I should have gotten a day-pass for him to come with me. I ended up paying top dollar for "Rosie," as we affectionately named our new addition to the garden.

It was around May when Mike and I lovingly put "Rosie" in the ground. She was about a foot tall. Pat, our expert on such things, insisted that it would never bloom the first year. "Oh yes it will," I confidently declared. "Not only that, I'll bet you that it will give forth a dozen roses." He assured me that I was wrong.

I laughed and said, "We'll just see. This child's intention is so strong, there is no way that God is going to let him down." We were both wrong. Rosie produced so many glorious roses that summer that I eventually lost count. I would wager to guess that it was somewhere around three dozen!

THE DIARY

Four days after the harvest party I got a call from my Aunt Jo (my mother's only sibling), another one of those relatives who never called just to chat. My mother had passed away that morning after years of slowly dying from emphysema and heart disease. I have to admit that I was relieved. She had been hooked to an oxygen machine like a puppy on a leash for the past ten years or so. She spent the vast majority of her days sitting at her kitchen table drawing or gazing out the window at the beautiful resort she lived in but could no longer enjoy.

My mother and I had had a rough go after my fifteen years absence from the family. But she had become one of my best friends in the last two years. I had called her frequently and we traded correspondence often. We even had a little art game going through the mail that we had played when I was a kid. I had visited her probably six times in the past eight years. The last time had been five months earlier.

I wanted to make sure that she felt loved by me and that we had some closure to our relationship. I didn't want to face any regrets after her death, so I had showed up on her doorstep for Mother's Day. I even had the taxi driver pull past the house so that she wouldn't know it was me until I walked through the door. She was thrilled!

We had a delightful visit. We played cards and did numerous art projects and talked about spirituality and death and dying. She had found great comfort in Bette Eddy's book, Embraced by the Light, and looked forward to meeting the angels and experiencing the after-life. She told me that she hoped she could be a better mother in her next life.

I confess that I had been expecting her to leave the planet ever since I had informed her that I was going to publish this exposé of our family. She couldn't handle reading it, but she had given me her blessings to publish it if I thought it would help others avoid the pain I had suffered. She also had agreed to illustrate it. But I didn't think she'd hang around to face the carnage in her super-rich community that had built a park in dedication to David Martin.

I landed in Texas thirty-six hours after my mother had taken her last breath. Jo was already there. My sister had never come back to the family and wanted nothing to do with any of it, and my brother was busy revamping Mom's house. I knew I was in for quite a ride with Sam.

During my Mother's Day visit, every time I had suggested we go find Sam Mom had gotten quite nervous. She finally mentioned that he didn't want anything to do with me because he didn't want me cramming my healthful lifestyle down his throat. She, too, was concerned about his alcoholism and smoking but had given up trying to talk to him about it.

Sam lived only a mile away, while I had traveled a thousand miles. I'm sure he hadn't missed a Mother's Day in twenty years, yet he never stopped by the house while I was there. So, you can imagine the stress I was feeling five months later as I walked into the house that I presumed now belonged to Sam, the executor of my mother's estate.

Jo beamed and greeted me warmly. Sam painted on a smile and uttered a polite hello. We chatted in the usual Martin manner — denial, as if nothing were wrong. Sam mentioned that there were people coming and I couldn't stay at the house. Before long he excused himself and left. He didn't really tell me what the plans were or where he wanted me to stay. He was just going to blow me off.

Jo had made herself at home in the master bedroom. In spite of Sam's comment, I parked in the guest bedroom, which was decorated in furniture that had been mine as a child.

After a couple of hours I couldn't stand the tension anymore — time to face the music — so I walked over to Sam's house. He looked like he'd seen a ghost when he answered the door.

I knew how to bond with my brother, though. I played dumb. "Aunt Jo is driving me crazy. Got a beer?" My drinking with him changed everything. He relaxed into the fun-loving being I had always remembered. As the evening wore on, his house filled up with his friends/ drinking buddies. Once they saw that Sam was embracing me, they were all quite warm. I was invited to move over to his house and drive my mother's car.

A few days later Sam and I each spoke at the memorial we hosted for our mother. Sam had created a darling handout that featured some of Mom's artwork and he had brought a few of her best pieces to display next to the coffin. Mom looked great in her pink suit (the only article of her clothing I had truly wanted when I was told that I could help myself to her wardrobe).

I spoke lovingly about what a supportive friend she had been and made jokes about her cheating at cards. I told the packed room of her friends that we had worked hard at creating a friendship after my returning to the family. I also told them that she had given me her blessings to publish my autobiography and that she had done the illustrations for it. I cried as I noted that it was the most courageous thing she'd ever done.

Sam delivered a glowing speech about what a generous, loving, mother, friend and philanthropist she had been. We hugged and cried when he turned the service over to the minister. I continued to cry as the singer blessed us with her rendition of the song I had picked out, my favorite, "In the Garden."

I had expected to be ostracized and even abused by this super-wealthy gathering of my parents' friends, as most of them knew I had caused my parents great pain by leaving the family. They swarmed me after the memorial. Amazingly they couldn't have been more supportive. They loved my speech and noted that my mother would have been thrilled with the service. Many of them wanted to know where they could purchase a copy of my book. I was in shock. I could barely put one foot in front of the other. I think Sam was equally overwhelmed by the warm reception I received.

My mother was to be buried next to my father in Indiana, where he had grown up. She hated that place but I don't think she really cared much where her remains would be parked. Sam bought two tickets and arranged for us to fly to the funeral a few days later. In the meantime, we barhopped, drank and reminisced about old times.

Sam's driver's license had expired and they wouldn't accept his credit card and my license so we couldn't rent a car upon landing in Chicago. We ended up taking a $200 cab ride, arriving an hour late for the funeral. As we were the only immediate family, they held the service for us. It was short and sweet. "Rest in peace...yadda yadda yadda," let's get out of here. We would be staying at our cousin Dick's house for the night and leaving the next afternoon by bus back to O'Hare.

I was pretty certain at this point that it was not going to be pretty when we got down to discussing the estate. One of Sam's friends had told me that he was planning on keeping the whole booty for himself. I was certain that Sam thought he deserved it all, since Paula and I had left the family and he had hung in there. My mother had gifted and/or lent me about $50,000 over the previous eight years and I could tell that he resented it, even though he had been gifted with at least ten times that and now had the whole estate in his hands.

The family was divided into two camps that evening at Dick's. The ladies were huddling with me and Sam was trying to squeeze an investment out of the men for the assisted living home he was building. The gals were on my side. They all knew what growing up with David Martin had been like and how abusive he could be. They felt that I was entitled to my share. I told them about the incest and my book for the first time. They weren't surprised. One of my cousins said that she had suspected sexual abuse as soon as she had learned that I had bailed out of the family. They were genuinely supportive. I felt fortified for the ordeal ahead.

The next day Sam flew back to Austin to return to Horseshoe Bay and I flew to Houston. My minister, Reverend Mary Manin Morrissey, was going to be speaking at the Unity church there and I thought I would gather my strength with her before confronting Sam about the estate. I bonded with a group of folks who had driven up from Galveston for the event. One of them, Roddy Webb, offered to put me up for a few days. I visited with Mary and some of the other speakers and then headed out with Roddy and his friends.

My stay with Roddy and his collection of bizarre animals was a whole life in itself. In my next book, Letters From Heaven, I will tell you about my close encounter with Roddy's vicious dog, the Rexagator. He re-earned his nickname during my stay.

It had been ten days since we had put my mother in the ground. I returned to Horseshoe Bay and decided that it was time to have "the talk" with Sam. My aunt had gotten a promise of her measly $10,000 inheritance and left town. I drove over to Sam's house in my mother's car. His secretary was within earshot in the office and he was at one of the many computers in the dining room. I sat down and hedged, "I'd like to talk to you about the estate."

He quietly responded, "I'm sorry, but they didn't leave you anything." I wasn't surprised. My father was apparently quite bitter towards me when he died. He was also a shrewd businessman. I had presumed that he had set up his will and the numerous trusts to make sure Paula and I never got a dime. I also suspected that even if my mother had wanted to share her wealth with us that she probably couldn't have, as Sam had been hovering over her and the money since David's death.

"Well, I'm not surprised. But it's not about them anymore. It's between you and me," I softly stated.

I can't remember his exact words but what I recall he said next was something like "You disowned them. I stayed in the family, so it's all mine."

The conversation began to escalate. I remember saying, "Hey, I spent the past eight years trying to have a relationship with her and it has not been easy. Besides, my disowning them is not the issue. The reason I left was to salvage my sanity. Anybody who spent eighteen years being abused by David Martin deserves a chunk of his money!"

Sam continued to contend that it was all his and that's that. After a little more ruckus I announced, "Well it's not going to go down this way!" and got up to leave.

He demanded the keys to the car and drove me back to Mom's house. Pat had flown in a few days before and was staying there with me along with the two women I had befriended, Debbie Camp and Delores Patty. They were in town trying to collect Debbie's divorce settlement and were having about as much success as I was.

Upon arriving at the house Sam insisted that we all pack our things and get out. I stated that I wasn't leaving. He called the police, who were all buddies of his. I raged at him in front of the four officers about the incest and the abortion I had lived through. Sam just hung his head. Pat tried to reason with him but got nowhere.

Sam even insisted that I leave the clothes and the books of Mom's that he had originally said I could take, stating again that it was all his. I screamed, "I have one of her bras on. Would you like me to take that off too?"

Debbie and Delores had split. The police literally put Pat and me on the street. We moved our bags over to the neighbors' driveway. Unfortunately, they were gone for the weekend. Debbie and Delores met us in town and moved into a motel. We had enough money left to last two days.

The interesting part of this whole mess had been Sam's drunken speech the night before. We had been at a party at his house. At one point Sam plunked down with me in the chair I was sitting in, put his arm around me and told me how much he loved me. He then proceeded to orate to his friends about what a great person I was and what great work I was doing. During our verbal judo the next day previous to the police action, he was telling me that I was a leech and needed to grow up and get a job.

To make a long story shorter, Pat went home and I set out to find an attorney who would help me fight for my share of the estate. No one knew exactly how much was really there, but the cousins and the neighbors estimated that it was definitely in the millions, possibly ten or more.

I had less than a hundred dollars left by the time Pat flew out. Debbie and Delores and I moved in with our friend, Alton Ray.

Debbie and Delores were nicknamed Thelma and Louise by the locals. Before long we were known as the Three Ds. I called Sam and told him that I didn't even have enough money to get out of town and that at the very least I wanted the $1600 I had borrowed for the privilege of attending my mother's memorial. I added that I was sure she had not wanted me to accrue a debt on her behalf. He agreed to write me a check. Like an idiot though, after picking up the check, I left him a message that I wasn't leaving and that I was going to sue the estate. He stopped payment on the check before I could get to the bank to cash it. I was as stupid as he was greedy!

The first order of business was to get my hands on both my parents' wills. I never suspected how big an impact reading these stacks of legalese would have on my life. After a few long weeks of anticipation, David's will arrived first. I was blown away. I had expected it to be a vicious document, cutting my sister and me off at the knees. It wasn't. I felt a lot of love and remorse from my father as I read his last will and testament. It basically stated that the bulk of the estate was to go to Sam, unless he was to die first, then it would be split equally between Paula and me. I was stunned for days. I felt a wonderful sense of peace and closure – perhaps my father had truly loved me after all.

The first attorney I met with warned me that my father's will was very tight – not much room for litigation. I was expecting a similar document from my mother. I could only hope for some loopholes that might appear on my behalf, or an attorney who had the chutzpa to sue the estate for childhood sexual abuse.

The impact my father's will had had on me was

nothing compared to the emotions that my mother's triggered. There it was, three-quarters of the way down the first page: "For the purpose of executing this last will and testament, consider that my daughters have predeceased me." I didn't need an attorney to translate it for me. It said, "Consider my daughters dead!" "You @#$! bitch!" I was livid. It wasn't the money that dug so deep. It was the viciousness of the phrase, especially considering our heart-felt visit five months earlier. Everybody tried to console me by insisting that it had been Sam's doing. I knew that he had wielded a lot of influence over my mother, but I also knew in my heart that this had probably been her choice. She had experienced a lot of pain over the fifteen years I was gone. She obviously was still harboring a great deal of resentment about it when she drafted this will eight years ago. Either she had never changed it or Sam had destroyed a more recent will after her death. I gave him the benefit of the doubt.

After reading my mother's will I knew it was time to give up. I talked to friends and family all over the country. I prayed about it. I meditated on it. I walked, ran and slept on it. The truth is, though, I knew the moment I read that phrase that it was over.

My spirituality is more important to me than anything else. What I wanted most of all was to find love in my heart. I found peace by believing that my mother had done this for a reason, even if it was subconscious and her surface feelings had been vindictive. The other ingredient that helped me find peace was my love for Sam. He had done some really ugly things to me over the past eight years, but no matter what, I always had this warm-fuzzy place in my heart for him. Somehow, as soon as I decided to let it go, I found that love for Sam again.

I called him and told him that I would rather have him in my life than the money, and that I was going to drop the suit. He said, "Works for me." We laughed and talked and arranged to get together for a drink before I left. He agreed to make sure that I got to the airport as I was wiped out financially.

He put me off every time we tried to get together and finally sent a friend who nearly made me miss my plane. His buddy beat me up energetically all the way to the airport. "How could you do this to Sam? He's such a great guy." That pissed me off but I managed to get over it. I continued to call, email and send birthday and Christmas cards for the next two years. Sam never would let me in. I finally realized that he will never be able to embrace me until he is willing to face the truth about his childhood. He can't have me and his denial too. I love you, Sam. I wish you peace.

It had been nearly ten weeks since my mother's death at this point. Debbie and Delores had been supporting me for the last eight weeks out of the measly settlement that Debbie had gotten from her well-to-do ex. Thanks, ladies, you're the best!

By the time I landed in Portland I was not only totally broke, but up to my eyeballs in debt. I mustered the energy to go back to seeking capital for our mission of promoting sacred foods. I told everyone that God would provide and I began to feel a certain essence of peace that I had never experienced before.

Within six weeks I was living in the most beautiful bed and breakfast in scenic northern Idaho that anyone could hope to visit. I was writing a business plan for a sustainable community which included the spacious bed and breakfast I was hosted in. The owner, Pam Dalby, was one of the most supportive people who has ever crossed my path. She let me run up the phone bill and turn the formal dining room into my office. She continually pumped me up with her belief in my ability.

Thanks, Pam!

One morning I was sleeping in my palatial, hand-carved wooden bed in the "John Wayne" room. It was the most macho room in the house, very suited to my aggressive personality. I had asked Pam to wake me up for church that morning. In the dream I was having, there was a window next to my bed. The curtains were blowing vigorously in the open window. When I saw the person approaching the window from the outside I thought it was Pam coming to wake me up for church.

When I looked closely out the window I saw that it was my mother standing there. The window was about waist high to her and she was standing on the ground barefooted. I was in shock in my dream. I said, "But, Mom, you're dead!" She looked about twenty years younger than the last time I had seen her and didn't have her trademark oxygen hose around her face.

She calmly asked, "Don't you know where I am?" I noted that my mother rarely went outside without her shoes on because she had suffered from corns on her feet all of her adult life. So I interpreted her question as meaning that she must be in her vision of heaven.

"I just dropped by to see if you are okay and if you have everything you need," she stated softly. I assured her that I was being well taken care of. I leaned towards the window to get a closer look at her. I was so incredulous at how real she appeared that I woke up with my heart leaping out of my chest. I cried for hours. I felt sure that this was an affirmation of my belief that she had sincerely had a loving reason for cutting me out of the will.

The next night I was reading in the book, Seth Speaks, I had bought from the second-hand store. It spoke of how people from the other side often visit us in our dreams — more validation.

During my visit in May, my mother and I had discussed that she should try and contact me after she passed on. We had even tried to come up with a symbol that I would recognize if she were to create it in my reality. It never occurred to us that she could just stroll into my consciousness as herself.

My mother gave me the opportunity to create my own legacy, instead of living off of hers. That is perhaps the greatest gift I have ever received. Thanks, Mom! Ten million wouldn't have served me as well.

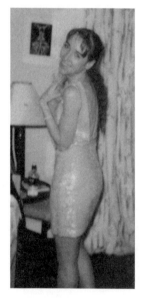

I'm not saying that my life is totally healed or that I have reached Christ-like enlightenment. I am just a work in progress and I am happy with my progress.

FOOD FOR THOUGHT...

Being able to believe that I have been sexually abused by my parents, or that they gave me an abortion, has been a journey, not an immediate truth that I embraced. The idea is so shocking and so gruesome, who wants to believe these things? During our two days or so at the house together after Mom's passing, Aunt Jo and I went through every nook and cranny hoping to find a pile of cash or diamonds that Sam hadn't already coveted. What we found was worth more to me than emeralds or hundred dollar bills.

Way in the back of a bottom shelf in the bathroom, I found a few belongings of my father's, including an old tattered little box. I didn't understand what the silver things in the box were at first, nor did I notice the writing on the side. Jo didn't know what they were either.

When I finally realized what it was, I was paralyzed. The items in the box were aluminum plugs that were each a little bigger than the last. In faded letters on the side of the box it said, "Cervical dilator." It had belonged to David's stepfather, who had been a doctor.

I can see my father keeping his stethoscope as a memento, or one of his white jackets, but a cervical dilator kit? My mother had always gotten the best medical care, her babies were never delivered at home. There is no reasonable explanation as to why he would have had this kit. I believe that God intended for me to find this ancient, supposedly worthless little box to help me validate my memories once and for all.

In short, Sam got the house, the money, the boat,

the stocks, the diamonds and the properties. I got a bra, a pair of boots, a $1600 debt, a diary and a cervical dilator kit. Believe it or not, I think I got the biggest haul from the estate. I got my power back from all of them!

JUST FOR FUN...

You are probably wondering about the title of this chapter. I can't wait to tell you about it!

At first, Sam had told me that I could have any of my mother's clothes that I wanted. I had invited her friends and Sam's to help themselves too. We gals were having a grand time in Mom's walk-in closet, as Mom had some nice stuff. Sam's friend Gail came out with this little black leather book in hand and said, "Look what I found." It was my mother's diary from her first year of college.

Before I tell you what was in the diary I have to give you a little background. My mother had made herself out to be the Virgin Mary herself. She had flat out told me that she had been a virgin when she married and was indicating that I should consider the same path. Fat chance!

One day I had come home from school when I was in the eighth grade and told her that we had been having a discussion in English about premarital sex. She slapped me across the face and barked, "What's to discuss? You don't do it!" She had mellowed some in her later years as Sam and I showed up with sweethearts in tow that we obviously were sleeping with but not married to. She even allowed us to sleep with them in her house after David died. But I still wasn't prepared for what I was about to learn about my dearly departed mother.

My Aunt Jo was there when the now infamous diary surfaced. After the ladies left with their selections, Jo and I sat down to devour this little peek into my mother's life. Jo had lived with my mother during this year of college. She had thought that my mother had majored in bridge. She was way off. Pat Martin, a.k.a. "The Virgin", drank and screwed her way through college. This diary would make Bill Clinton's autobiography look like a Sesame Street primer.

I had to stop Jo every hour or so and make sure her heart was still ticking. She would roar and laugh and rant as she worked her way through the diary. She knew many of these people and was delightfully taking notes with the intent of contacting some of them when she got back home. In the back of the little black book there were almost two hundred names of men, with codes and symbols next to their names. Remember, this was one year of my mother's college life. It wasn't quite clear from the daily dialogues whether she was sleeping with all these men or just teasing them.

Aunt Jo told me a story, though, of a night when my grandmother had confronted my mother with a semen-soaked dress. We knew she had slept with that guy, so we looked him up in the back and noted the symbols next to his name and broke the code. "Mom, you were a naughty, naughty girl. I bet you're wishing that I had predeceased you now!" I love her even more since reading the diary, though. The truth really can set us free. It is shame, and secrets, that keep us in shackles.

I hope that my journey towards personal freedom has been entertaining and/or enlightening for you. Being conscious of what I consume continues to be the fastest path to bliss that I have discovered thus far. And when I add a positive attitude and faith and love to that equation, I find myself in Heaven on Earth. I give into my overwhelm and my addictions at times, but I am informed about the affects on me, leaping back into the garden faster each time. I know that I can choose to live in either Heaven or Hell. I choose Heaven.

Faith creates!

Well, friends, thanks for listening and for investing in my mission. There is still way more to tell, though. I hope you'll look for my next book, *Letters From Heaven*, out soon. Please visit me at:

www.eatingmywaytoheaven.com

God Bless You and Bon Appetit!

Eating My Way to Heaven

Epilogue

Well, well, well. Here we are again. Four more years have passed since I wrote the last chapter. And, once again, I have packed a lifetime's worth of trauma, drama and excitement into those forty-eight months. But I've given you plenty of bang for your buck already, so you'll have to buy my next book, **Letters From Heaven**, to read about it.

Here's a little teaser, however:

There were many significant events I had to leave out of my life story in order to be able to lift the manuscript, as I have lived rather large. Interestingly, although I chronicled most of my major injuries and ailments I didn't chose to tell you that I had descended into menopause at age thirty-eight. I was being knocked off my feet by vicious hot flashes, my periods were just about non-existent and my emotions were all over the map. The Natural Health Practitioner I was working with told me that it was not reversible but that there were some remedies that would make the ride more comfortable for me.

Apparently though, the *Eating My Way to Heaven* diet healed my fertility too. Meet my son, Ezekiel, conceived naturally and born vaginally on March 9th, 2004. I was 47 years old at the time, and I have energy to burn, even as a full-time mom who runs her business in the middle of the night while her darling baby sleeps.

So I guess the reason I couldn't get this book on the market until now is because God had more Heaven for me, I just had to step back in hell for a while in order to receive it and appreciate it. Make no mistake. I could not be more blessed or more grateful for the beautiful life that my choices and my faith have created. Thank You God!

Faith Creates!

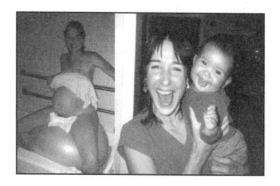